MEASURING THE IMPACT OF INTERPROFESSIONAL EDUCATION ON COLLABORATIVE PRACTICE AND PATIENT OUTCOMES

Committee on Measuring the Impact of Interprofessional Education on Collaborative Practice and Patient Outcomes

Board on Global Health

INSTITUTE OF MEDICINE
OF THE NATIONAL ACADEMIES

THE NATIONAL ACADEMIES PRESS
Washington, D.C.
www.nap.edu

THE NATIONAL ACADEMIES PRESS   500 Fifth Street, NW   Washington, DC 20001

NOTICE: The project that is the subject of this report was approved by the Governing Board of the National Research Council, whose members are drawn from the councils of the National Academy of Sciences, the National Academy of Engineering, and the Institute of Medicine. The members of the committee responsible for the report were chosen for their special competences and with regard for appropriate balance.

This activity was supported by contracts between the National Academy of Sciences and the Academic Consortium for Complementary and Alternative Health Care, the Academy of Nutrition and Dietetics, the Accreditation Council for Graduate Medical Education, the Aetna Foundation, the Alliance for Continuing Education in the Health Professions, the American Academy of Family Physicians, the American Academy of Nursing, the American Association of Colleges of Nursing, the American Association of Colleges of Osteopathic Medicine, the American Association of Colleges of Pharmacy, the American Association of Nurse Anesthetists, the American Association of Nurse Practitioners, the American Board of Family Medicine, the American Board of Internal Medicine, the American College of Nurse-Midwives, the American Congress of Obstetricians and Gynecologists/American Board of Obstetrics and Gynecology, the American Council of Academic Physical Therapy, the American Dental Education Association, the American Medical Association, the American Occupational Therapy Association, the American Psychological Association, the American Society for Nutrition, the American Speech–Language–Hearing Association, the Association of American Medical Colleges, the Association of American Veterinary Medical Colleges, the Association of Schools and Colleges of Optometry, the Association of Schools and Programs of Public Health, the Association of Schools of the Allied Health Professions, the Atlantic Philanthropies, the China Medical Board, the Council of Academic Programs in Communication Sciences and Disorders, the Council on Social Work Education, Ghent University, the Josiah Macy Jr. Foundation, Kaiser Permanente, the National Academies of Practice, the National Association of Social Workers, the National Board for Certified Counselors, Inc. and Affiliates, the National Board of Medical Examiners, the National League for Nursing, the Office of Academic Affiliations of the Veterans Health Administration, the Organization of Associate Degree Nursing, the Physician Assistant Education Association, the Robert Wood Johnson Foundation, the Society for Simulation in Healthcare, the Uniformed Services University of the Health Sciences, and the University of Toronto. Any opinions, findings, conclusions, or recommendations expressed in this publication are those of the authors and do not necessarily reflect the views of the organizations or agencies that provided support for the project.

International Standard Book Number-13:   978-0-309-37282-4
International Standard Book Number-10:   0-309-37282-8

Additional copies of this workshop summary are available for sale from the National Academies Press, 500 Fifth Street, NW, Keck 360, Washington, DC 20001; (800) 624-6242 or (202) 334-3313; http://www.nap.edu.

For more information about the Institute of Medicine, visit the IOM home page at: http://iom.nationalacademies.org.

The serpent has been a symbol of long life, healing, and knowledge among almost all cultures and religions since the beginning of recorded history. The serpent adopted as a logotype by the Institute of Medicine is a relief carving from ancient Greece, now held by the Staatliche Museen in Berlin.

Cover photo © 2015 Diane Melms, *Behold*. Size 76 × 32 inches. Fabric hand-dyed by artist, line patterns printed on fabric with textile paint using a mono-print technique, shapes cut freehand with rotary cutter, machine pieced, layered with batting and machine quilted. Documentation of the creation of this piece is on the SAQA website: http://www.saqa.com/media/file/SPal/MelmsBinder1.pdf.

Suggested citation: IOM (Institute of Medicine). 2015. *Measuring the impact of interprofessional education on collaborative practice and patient outcomes*. Washington, DC: The National Academies Press.

*"Knowing is not enough; we must apply.
Willing is not enough; we must do."*
—Goethe

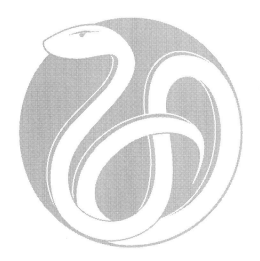

INSTITUTE OF MEDICINE
OF THE NATIONAL ACADEMIES

Advising the Nation. Improving Health.

THE NATIONAL ACADEMIES
Advisers to the Nation on Science, Engineering, and Medicine

The **National Academy of Sciences** is a private, nonprofit, self-perpetuating society of distinguished scholars engaged in scientific and engineering research, dedicated to the furtherance of science and technology and to their use for the general welfare. Upon the authority of the charter granted to it by the Congress in 1863, the Academy has a mandate that requires it to advise the federal government on scientific and technical matters. Dr. Ralph J. Cicerone is president of the National Academy of Sciences.

The **National Academy of Engineering** was established in 1964, under the charter of the National Academy of Sciences, as a parallel organization of outstanding engineers. It is autonomous in its administration and in the selection of its members, sharing with the National Academy of Sciences the responsibility for advising the federal government. The National Academy of Engineering also sponsors engineering programs aimed at meeting national needs, encourages education and research, and recognizes the superior achievements of engineers. Dr. C. D. Mote, Jr., is president of the National Academy of Engineering.

The **Institute of Medicine** was established in 1970 by the National Academy of Sciences to secure the services of eminent members of appropriate professions in the examination of policy matters pertaining to the health of the public. The Institute acts under the responsibility given to the National Academy of Sciences by its congressional charter to be an adviser to the federal government and, upon its own initiative, to identify issues of medical care, research, and education. Dr. Victor J. Dzau is president of the Institute of Medicine.

The **National Research Council** was organized by the National Academy of Sciences in 1916 to associate the broad community of science and technology with the Academy's purposes of furthering knowledge and advising the federal government. Functioning in accordance with general policies determined by the Academy, the Council has become the principal operating agency of both the National Academy of Sciences and the National Academy of Engineering in providing services to the government, the public, and the scientific and engineering communities. The Council is administered jointly by both Academies and the Institute of Medicine. Dr. Ralph J. Cicerone and Dr. C. D. Mote, Jr., are chair and vice chair, respectively, of the National Research Council.

www.national-academies.org

COMMITTEE ON MEASURING THE IMPACT OF INTERPROFESSIONAL EDUCATION ON COLLABORATIVE PRACTICE AND PATIENT OUTCOMES

MALCOLM COX (*Chair*), Adjunct Professor, Perelman School of Medicine, University of Pennsylvania

BARBARA F. BRANDT, Director, National Center for Interprofessional Practice and Education, University of Minnesota

JANICE PALAGANAS, Director of Educational Innovation and Development, Center for Medical Simulation, Massachusetts General Hospital, Harvard Medical School

SCOTT REEVES, Professor in Interprofessional Research, Centre for Health and Social Care Research, Kingston University and St George's, University of London

ALBERT W. WU, Professor and Director, Center for Health Services and Outcomes Research, Johns Hopkins Bloomberg School of Public Health

BRENDA ZIERLER, Co-Director, Center for Health Sciences Interprofessional Education, Practice and Research, University of Washington

Consultants

VALENTINA L. BRASHERS, Founding Co-Director of the Center for ASPIRE, University of Virginia

MAY NAWAL LUTFIYYA, Senior Research Scientist, National Center for Interprofessional Practice and Education

NELSON SEWANKAMBO, Principal and Professor, Makerere University College of Health Sciences

RONA BRIERE, Consultant Editor

IOM Staff

PATRICIA A. CUFF, Senior Program Officer
MEGAN M. PEREZ, Research Associate
BRIDGET CALLAGHAN, Research Assistant (from January 2015)
AEYSHA CHAUDRY, Intern
CHRISTIE BELL, Financial Officer (from January 2015)
ROSALIND GOMES, Financial Associate (until December 2014)
PATRICK W. KELLEY, Senior Board Director, Board on Global Health

Reviewers

This report has been reviewed in draft form by individuals chosen for their diverse perspectives and technical expertise, in accordance with procedures approved by the National Research Council's Report Review Committee. The purpose of this independent review is to provide candid and critical comments that will assist the institution in making its published report as sound as possible and to ensure that the report meets institutional standards for objectivity, evidence, and responsiveness to the study charge. The review comments and draft manuscript remain confidential to protect the integrity of the deliberative process. We wish to thank the following individuals for their review of this report:

HUGH BARR, University of Westminster, UK
MOLLY COOKE, University of California, San Francisco
SUSAN HASSMILLER, Robert Wood Johnson Foundation
LANA SUE KAʻOPUA, University of Hawaiʻi-Mānoa
EDUARDO SALAS, University of Central Florida
JILL THISTLETHWAITE, University of Technology Sydney, Australia
MERRICK ZWARENSTEIN, Western University, London, Ontario

Although the reviewers listed above provided many constructive comments and suggestions, they were not asked to endorse the report's conclusions or recommendations, nor did they see the final draft of the report before its release. The review of this report was overseen by **CAROL PEARL HERBERT,** University of British Columbia, Vancouver, BC, and Western University, London, Ontario, and **SUSAN J. CURRY,** University of Iowa.

Appointed by the Institute of Medicine and the National Research Council, they were responsible for making certain that an independent examination of this report was carried out in accordance with institutional procedures and that all review comments were carefully considered. Responsibility for the final content of this report rests entirely with the authoring committee and the institution.

Contents

Glossary[1]

Collaboration is an active and ongoing partnership, often involving people from diverse backgrounds who work together to solve problems, provide services, and enhance outcomes.

Collaborative patient-centered practice is a type of arrangement designed to promote the participation of patients and their families within a context of collaborative practice.

Continuing education encompasses all learning (e.g., formal, informal, workplace, serendipitous) that enhances understanding and improves patient care.

Continuing professional development is self-directed learning that ensures continuing professional competence throughout one's health professional career.

Entrustable professional activities is a "concept that allows faculty to make competency-based decisions on the level of supervision required by trainees." (ten Cate, 2013).

---

[1] Unless otherwise noted, these definitions are based on the work of Barr et al. (2005) and Reeves et al. (2010). Note that this glossary includes only terms that appear in the report. The committee recognizes that many definitions for these terms exist and that some definitions evolve over time.

Evaluation refers to the systematic gathering and interpretation of evidence enabling judgment of effectiveness and value and promoting improvement. Evaluations can have either formative or summative elements or both.

Interprofessional collaboration is a type of interprofessional work involving various health and social care professionals who come together regularly to solve problems, provide services, and enhance health outcomes.

Interprofessional education "occurs when two or more professions learn with, about, and from each other to enable effective collaboration and improve health outcomes." (WHO, 2010)

Interprofessional learning is learning arising from interaction involving members or students of two or more professions. It may be a product of *interprofessional education,* or it may occur spontaneously in the workplace or in education settings and therefore be serendipitous.

Interprofessional teamwork is a type of work involving different health or social care professionals who share a team identity and work together closely in an integrated and interdependent manner to solve problems, deliver services, and enhance health outcomes.

One Health recognizes that the health of humans, animals, and ecosystems is interconnected.

Profession refers to an occupation or career that requires considerable training and specialized study.

Quality improvement is defined by Batalden and Davidoff (2007, p. 2) as "the combined and unceasing efforts of everyone—healthcare professionals, patients and their families, researchers, payers, planners and educators—to make the changes that will lead to better patient outcomes (health), better system performance (care) and better professional development."

Realist evaluation is a method developed by Pawson and Tilley (1997) for analyzing the social context in which an intervention does or does not achieve its intended outcome.

Team-based care is an approach to health care whereby a group of people work together to accomplish a common goal, solve a problem, or achieve a specified result.

Workplace learning is different from formal educational activities, and can be viewed as untapped opportunities for learning and change that are part of everyday practice and often go unrecognized as "learning."

REFERENCES

Barr, H., I. Koppel, S. Reeves, M. Hammick, and D. Freeth. 2005. *Effective interprofessional education: Argument, assumption, and evidence.* Oxford and Malden: Blackwell Publishing.

Batalden, P. B., and F. Davidoff. 2007. What is "quality improvement" and how can it transform healthcare? *Quality & Safety in Health Care* 16(1):2-3.

Pawson, R., and N. Tilley. 1997. *Realistic evaluation.* London: Sage Publications.

Reeves, S., S. Lewin, S. Espin, and M. Zwarenstein. 2010. *Interprofessional teamwork for health and social care.* London: Wiley-Blackwell.

ten Cate, O. 2013. Nuts and bolts of entrustable professional activities. *Journal of Graduate Medical Education* 5(1):157-158.

WHO (World Health Organization). 2010. *Framework for action on interprofessional education and collaborative practice.* Geneva: WHO.

Preface

In 2002, the Institute of Medicine (IOM) convened a summit of diverse stakeholders who made the case for reforming health professions education to improve the quality and safety of health care. While many of their recommendations remain relevant today, much has changed over the past decade, necessitating new thinking. Innovators at that time stressed the importance of "patient-centered care," while today they think of patients as partners in health promotion and health care delivery. Patients are integral members of the care team, not solely patients to be treated, and the team is recognized as comprising a variety of health professionals. This changed thinking is the culmination of many social, economic, and technological factors that are transforming the world and forcing the fields of both health care and education to rethink long-established organizational models.

This report examines the evidence linking interprofessional education to patient and health system outcomes and provides general guidance on approaches to strengthening this evidence base in the future. Although this was the study committee's primary focus, however, it became clear early in the committee's deliberations that there are two essential prerequisites for the successful completion of this important task. First, efforts to reform education of the health care workforce and redesign practice in the health care system need to be better aligned. Because change in one of these interacting systems inevitably influences the other, efforts to improve interprofessional education or collaborative practice independently have fallen short. Second, widespread adoption of a model of interprofessional education across the learning continuum is urgently needed. An ideal model would retain the tenets of professional identity formation while providing robust opportunities for interprofessional education and collaborative care. Such a model also would differentiate between learning outcomes per se and the individual, population, and system outcomes that provide the ultimate rationale for ongoing investment in health professions education. And it would take into account the many enabling or interfering influences on learning and these more distal outcomes.

The committee hopes its appraisal of the evidence linking interprofessional education to enhanced health and system outcomes will catalyze additional studies that provide a stronger rationale for interprofessional education and collaborative care than is presently available. The committee likewise hopes that the presentation of an outcomes-based model of interprofessional education will stimulate the model's further refinement and thereby promote improvements in study design and execution.

Once tested, such a model could be adapted to fit the particular needs of higher- and lower-resource settings around the globe. It is no longer acceptable to think of either health or education in isolation. The final model must accommodate the reality of today's globalized community. It is through this lens that this report is intended to be read. In essence, the committee asks readers of this report to consider how all health professionals and all countries might learn and work together to maximize the health and well-being of individuals and populations around the world.

Malcolm Cox, *Chair*
Committee on Measuring the Impact of
Interprofessional Education on Collaborative
Practice and Patient Outcomes

Summary

Over the past half century, there have been ebbs and flows of interest in linking what is now called *interprofessional education* (IPE) with interprofessional collaboration and team-based care. As a result, a commitment to designing, implementing, and evaluating IPE curricula also has come in and out of favor. Since the mid-2000s, concerns about the quality and cost of health care, limited access to care for some groups and populations, and patient safety, together with increasing interest in transforming health professions education, have stimulated a resurgence of interest in IPE as a viable approach to developing interprofessional competencies for effective collaborative practice (IOM, 2000, 2001). Today, however, as contemporary health care approaches have become more outcomes-based, so have the questions raised about the impact and effectiveness of IPE (Cerra and Brandt, 2011; IPEC, 2011). Whereas considerable research has focused on student learning, only recently have researchers begun to look beyond the classroom and beyond learning outcomes for the impact of IPE on such issues as patient safety, patient and provider satisfaction, quality of care, health promotion, population health, and the cost of care (Moore et al., 2009; Walsh et al., 2014).

STUDY CHARGE

In this context, the Institute of Medicine (IOM) convened the Committee on Measuring the Impact of Interprofessional Education on Collaborative Practice and Patient Outcomes. The committee was charged to "analyze the available data and information to determine the best methods

1

for measuring the impact of interprofessional education (IPE) on specific aspects of health care delivery and the functioning of health care systems." The committee's charge required moving beyond examining the impact of IPE on learners' knowledge, skills, and attitudes to focus on the link between IPE and performance in practice, including the impact of IPE on patient and population health and health care delivery system outcomes. Learning has been defined as the act of "developing knowledge, skills or new insights, bringing about a change in understanding, perspective, or the way something is done or acted upon" (Nisbet et al., 2013, p. 469). Therefore, how a professional masters knowledge as an individual or as part of an interprofessional team, group, or network; develops new skills; modifies attitudes and behaviors; and achieves competence and expertise over time all impact these outcomes.

The particular setting within which learning occurs also is vitally important (Bridges et al., 2011; Oandasan and Reeves, 2005; Salas and Rosen, 2013; WHO, 2010). Given the rapidity with which health care around the world is changing, the committee quickly realized the need to reconsider the existing paradigm of how, where, and with whom health professions learning takes place. A central tenet of this shift in perspective is the need to recognize the vital role of the direct involvement of patients, families, and communities in the education-to-practice continuum to help ensure that education, training, and professional development are designed in ways that have a positive impact on health. Therefore, the desired outcome is not just improving learning but improving the health of individuals and populations and enhancing the responsiveness of health systems to such nonhealth dimensions as respect for patients and families, consumer satisfaction, and the affordability of health care for all.

Another question the committee had to confront is whether it is possible to evaluate the impact of any health professions education intervention on improving health or system outcomes given the degree to which confounding variables can obscure the evaluation results. Such variables can be in the form of enabling or interfering factors in such areas as professional or institutional culture and workforce or financing policy.

ADDRESSING THE GAPS

In reviewing the IPE literature, it became apparent that it is possible to link the learning process with downstream person-, population-, or system-directed outcomes provided that thoughtful, collaborative, and well-designed studies are intentionally targeted to answering such questions. Despite accumulating data, however, the committee identified numerous gaps in the evidence linking IPE to patient, population, and system outcomes.

In light of these gaps, the committee found it necessary to highlight four areas that, if addressed, would lay a strong foundation for evaluating the impact of IPE on collaborative practice and patient, population, and system outcomes: (1) more closely aligning the education and health care delivery systems, (2) developing a conceptual framework for measuring the impact of IPE, (3) strengthening the evidence base for IPE, and (4) linking IPE with changes in collaborative behavior.

Alignment of Education and Health Care Delivery Systems

Coordinated planning among educators, health system leaders, and policy makers is a prerequisite to creating an optimal learning environment and an effective health workforce (Cox and Naylor, 2013). To this end, educators need to be cognizant of health system redesign efforts, while health system leaders need to recognize the realities of educating and training a competent health workforce. Joint planning is especially important when health systems are undergoing rapid changes, as they are across much of the world today (Coker et al., 2008). IPE is particularly affected by the need for joint planning because the practice environment is where much of the imprinting of such concepts as collaboration and effective teamwork takes place. Despite calls for greater alignment, however, education reform is rarely well integrated with health system redesign (Cox and Naylor, 2013; Earnest and Brandt, 2014; Frenk et al., 2010; Ricketts and Fraher, 2013; WHO, 2010, 2011). Accountability for workforce and health outcomes often is dispersed among academic health centers and health care networks (Ovseiko et al., 2014). Possible exceptions include the rare cases in which ministries of education and health work together on individual initiatives (Booth, 2014; Frenk et al., 2010; MOH, 2014). Even in these cases, however, collaboration tends to be restricted to a single health profession.

Conclusion 1. Without a purposeful and more comprehensive system of engagement between the education and health care delivery systems, evaluating the impact of IPE interventions on health and system outcomes will be difficult.

Such engagement will require the active participation of the major health professions and the health system venues within which their students and practitioners learn together. It would be further enabled if individuals and organizations responsible for overseeing health professions education and health care delivery (including patient, population, and system outcomes) were to align and assume joint accountability for IPE across the lifelong learning continuum.

A Conceptual Framework for Measuring the Impact of IPE

Following an extensive literature search for interprofessional models of learning, the committee determined that no such models sufficiently incorporate all of the components needed to guide future studies effectively. The committee therefore developed a conceptual model that encompasses the education-to-practice continuum, a broad array of learning- and health-related outcomes, and major enabling and interfering factors. The committee puts forth this model with the understanding that it will need to be tested empirically and may need to be adapted to the particular settings in which it is applied. For example, educational structures and terminology differ considerably around the world, and the model may need to be modified to suit local or national conditions. However, the model's overarching concepts—a learning continuum, learning- and health-related outcomes, and major enabling and interfering factors—would remain.

Adoption of a conceptual model of IPE to guide future study designs would focus related research and evaluations on patient, population, or system outcomes that go beyond learning and testing of team function. Visualizing the entire IPE process illuminates the different environments where IPE exists, as well as the importance of aligning education and practice.

> *Conclusion 2. Having a comprehensive conceptual model would greatly enhance the description and purpose of IPE interventions and their potential impact. Such a model would provide a consistent taxonomy and framework for strengthening the evidence base linking IPE with health and system outcomes.*

Without such a framework, evaluating the impact of IPE on health and system outcomes will be difficult and perhaps impossible. If the individuals and organizations responsible for promoting, overseeing, and evaluating IPE were to address this gap—assuming joint accountability for the development of a consistent taxonomy and comprehensive conceptual framework that accurately describe IPE and all its outcomes—more systematic and robust research would likely be produced.

A Stronger Evidence Base

A comprehensive literature search revealed a dearth of robust studies specifically designed to better link IPE with changes in collaborative behavior or answer key questions about the effectiveness of IPE in improving health and system outcomes. The lack of a well-defined relationship between IPE and patient and population health and health care delivery system outcomes is due in part to the complexity of the learning and practice environments. It is difficult to generate this evidence in well-resourced settings, but even more difficult in parts of the world with fewer research and data resources (Price, 2005; Weaver et al., 2011).

Efforts to generate this evidence are further hindered by the relatively long lag time between education interventions and patient, population, and system outcomes; the lack of a commonly agreed-upon taxonomy and conceptual model linking education interventions to specific outcomes; and inconsistencies in study designs and methods and a lack of full reporting on the methods employed, which reduce the applicability and generalizability of many IPE study findings (Abu-Rish et al., 2012; Cooper et al., 2001; Olson and Bialocerkowski, 2014; Reeves et al., 2011, 2013; Remington et al., 2006; Salas et al., 2008a; Weaver et al., 2010; Zwarenstein et al., 2009).

There also are a plethora of enabling and interfering factors that directly or indirectly impact outcomes and program evaluation. Diverse and often opaque payment structures and differences in professional and organizational cultures generate obstacles to innovative workforce arrangements, thereby impeding interprofessional work. On the other hand, positive changes in workforce and financing policies could enable more effective collaboration and foster more robust evaluation.

Conclusion 3. More purposeful, well-designed, and thoughtfully reported studies are needed to answer key questions about the effectiveness of IPE in improving performance in practice and health and system outcomes.

Linking IPE with Changes in Collaborative Behavior

An essential intermediate step in linking IPE with health and system outcomes is enhanced collaborative behavior and performance in practice. While considerable attention has been focused on developing measures of interprofessional collaboration (CIHC, 2012; McDonald et al., 2014; National Center for Interprofessional Practice and Education, 2013; Reeves et al., 2010; Schmitz and Cullen, 2015), no such measures have as yet been broadly accepted or adopted (Clifton, 2006; Hammick et al., 2007; Thannhauser et al., 2010). In fact, the strong contextual dependence of presently available measures (Valentine et al., 2015; WHO, 2013) limits their application beyond a single study or small group of studies. To address this deficiency the committee makes the following recommendation:

Recommendation 1: Interprofessional stakeholders, funders, and policy makers should commit resources to a coordinated series of well-designed studies of the association between interprofessional education and collaborative behavior, including teamwork and performance in

practice. These studies should be focused on developing broad consensus on how to measure interprofessional collaboration effectively across a range of learning environments, patient populations, and practice settings.

These studies could employ different approaches that might include developing instruments and testing their reliability, validity, and usefulness specific to collaborative practice; conducting head-to-head comparisons of existing instruments within particular contexts; and extending the validation process for an existing "best-in-class" instrument to additional professions, learning environments, patient populations, health care settings, and countries. At a minimum, however, these studies should take into account the intended learner outcomes in the three major components of the education continuum—foundational education, graduate education, and continuing professional development. Therefore, each such study should clearly define the intermediate (learner) and more distal (health and system) outcome target(s).

Addressing these four gaps will entail giving IPE greater priority by forming partnerships among the education, practice, and research communities to design studies that are relevant to individual, population, and health system outcomes. Engaging accreditors, policy makers, and funders in the process could provide additional resources for establishing more robust partnerships. Only by bringing all these constituencies together will a series of well-designed studies emerge.

IMPROVING RESEARCH METHODOLOGIES

Understanding the full complexity of IPE and the education and health care delivery systems within which it resides is critical for designing studies to measure the impact of IPE on individual, population, and health system outcomes. Given this complexity, the use of a single type of research method alone may generate findings that fail to provide sufficient detail and context to be informative. IPE research would gain in stature from the adoption of a mixed-methods approach that combines focused quantitative and qualitative data to yield insight into the "what" and "how" of an IPE intervention/activity and its outcomes. Such an approach has been shown to be particularly useful for exploring the perceptions of both individuals and society regarding issues of quality of care and patient safety (Curry et al., 2009; De Lisle, 2011).

The committee recognizes the value of using a variety of data sources and methods for measuring the impact of IPE, including large data sets (i.e., "big data") for exploring potential relationships among variables. Similarly, the committee acknowledges the reality that demonstrating a return on investment will generally be necessary to spur greater financial investments in IPE. This is where alignment between the education and health care delivery systems becomes critical so that both the academic partner (creating the IPE intervention) and the health care delivery system partner (hosting the intervention and showcasing its outcomes) are working together. In this regard, policy makers, regulatory agencies, accrediting bodies, and professional organizations that oversee or encourage collaborative practice might provide additional incentives for programs and organizations to better align IPE with collaborative practice so that the potential long-term savings in health care can be evaluated.

Another issue identified by the committee is that a majority of IPE research is conducted by individual educators working alone who may not have evaluation expertise or time and resources to conduct the protocols required to address the key questions in the field. In the absence of robust research designs, there is a distinct risk that future studies testing the impact of IPE on health and system outcomes will continue to be unknowingly biased, underpowered to measure true differences, and not generalizable across different systems. These problems could be overcome by teams of individuals with complementary expertise, including an educational evaluator, a health services researcher, and an economist, in addition to educators and others engaged in IPE.

Based on the evidence and the committee's expert opinion, it is apparent that using either quantitative or qualitative methods alone will limit the ability of investigators in both developed and developing countries to produce high-quality studies linking IPE with patient, population, and health system outcomes. The committee therefore makes the following recommendation:

> **Recommendation 2: Health professions educators and academic and health system leaders should adopt a mixed-methods research approach for evaluating the impact of interprofessional education (IPE) on health and system outcomes. When possible, such studies should include an economic analysis and be carried out by teams of experts that include educational evaluators, health services researchers, and economists, along with educators and others engaged in IPE.**

Once best practices for designing, implementing, and evaluating IPE outcomes have been established, disseminating them widely through detailed reporting or publishing can strengthen the evidence base and help guide future studies linking IPE to outcomes. Such studies should include those focused on eliciting in-depth patient, family, and caregiver experiences of interprofessional collaborative practice. In the meantime, the committee has developed an outline of the key elements of a potential program for research connecting IPE to health and system outcomes for further consideration by educators, health care delivery system leaders, and policy makers.

CLOSING REMARKS

Although there is a widespread and growing belief that IPE may improve interprofessional collaboration, promote team-based health care delivery, and enhance personal and population health, definitive evidence linking IPE to desirable intermediate and final outcomes does not yet exist. This report identifies and analyzes the major challenges to closing this evidence gap and offers a range of strategies for overcoming barriers that limit the establishment of a clear linkage between IPE and improved health and system outcomes.

The committee reached three major conclusions and formulated two recommendations that collectively are aimed at elevating the profile of IPE in a rapidly changing world. The committee hopes this report will shed additional light on the value of collaboration between educators and practitioners and patients, families, and communities, as well as all those who come together in working to improve lives through treatment and palliation, disease prevention, and wellness interventions. As with other forms of health professions education, only through the publication of rigorously designed studies can the potential impact of IPE on health and health care be fully realized.

REFERENCES

Abu-Rish, E., S. Kim, L. Choe, L. Varpio, E. Malik, A. A. White, K. Craddick, K. Blondon, L. Robins, P. Nagasawa, A. Thigpen, L. L. Chen, J. Rich, and B. Zierler. 2012. Current trends in interprofessional education of health sciences students: A literature review. *Journal of Interprofessional Care* 26(6):444-451.

Booth, D. 2014. *Remarks by U.S. Ambassador Donald Booth at the inauguration of the new medical education initiative Ambo University.* http://ethiopia.usembassy.gov/latest_embassy_news/remarks/remarks-by-u.s.-ambassador-donald-booth-on-inauguration-of-the-new-medical-education-initiative-ambo-university (accessed January 12, 2015).

Bridges, D. R., R. A. Davidson, P. S. Odegard, I. V. Maki, and J. Tomkowiak. 2011. Interprofessional collaboration: Three best practice models of interprofessional education. *Medical Education Online* 16(6035):1-10.

Cerra, F., and B. F. Brandt. 2011. Renewed focus in the United States links interprofessional education with redesigning health care. *Journal of Interprofessional Care* 25(6):394-396.

CIHC (Canadian Interprofessional Health Collaborative). 2012. *An inventory of quantitative tools measuring interprofessional education and collaborative practice outcomes.* Vancouver, BC: CIHC.

Clifton, M., C. Dale, and C. Bradshaw. 2006. *The impact and effectiveness of inter-professional education in primary care: An RCN literature review.* London, England: Royal College of Nursing. https://www.rcn.org.uk/__data/assets/pdf_file/0004/78718/003091.pdf (accessed March 17, 2015).

Coker, R., R. A. Atun, and M. McKee. 2008. *Health systems and the challenge of communicable diseases: Experiences from Europe and Latin America, European Observatory on Health Systems and Policies Series.* Maidenhead and New York: McGraw-Hill Education.

Cooper, H., C. Carlisle, T. Gibbs, and C. Watkins. 2001. Developing an evidence base for inter-disciplinary learning: A systematic review. *Journal of Advanced Nursing* 35(2):228-237.

Cox, M., and M. Naylor. 2013. *Transforming patient care: Aligning interprofessional education with clinical practice redesign*. Proceedings of a Conference sponsored by the Josiah Macy Jr. Foundation in January 2013. New York: Josiah Macy Jr. Foundation. http://macyfoundation.org/docs/macy_pubs/JMF_TransformingPatientCare_Jan2013Conference_fin_Web.pdf (accessed March 17, 2014).

Curry, L. A., I. M. Nembhard, and E. H. Bradley. 2009. Qualitative and mixed methods provide unique contributions to outcomes research. *Circulation* 119(10):1442-1452.

De Lisle, J. 2011. The benefits and challenges of mixing methods and methodologies: Lessons learnt from implementing qualitatively led mixed methods research designs in Trinidad and Tobago. *Caribbean Curriculum* 18:87-120.

Earnest, M., and B. Brandt. 2014. Aligning practice redesign and interprofessional education to advance triple aim outcomes. *Journal of Interprofessional Care* 28(6):497-500.

Frenk, J., L. Chen, Z. A. Bhutta, J. Cohen, N. Crisp, T. Evans, H. Fineberg, P. Garcia, Y. Ke, P. Kelley, B. Kistnasamy, A. Meleis, D. Naylor, A. Pablos-Mendez, S. Reddy, S. Scrimshaw, J. Sepulveda, D. Serwadda, and H. Zurayk. 2010. Health professionals for a new century: Transforming education to strengthen health systems in an interdependent world. *Lancet* 376(9756):1923-1958.

Hammick, M., D. Freeth, I. Koppel, S. Reeves, and H. Barr. 2007. A best evidence systematic review of interprofessional education: BEME guide no. 9. *Medical Teacher* 29(8):735-751.

IOM (Institute of Medicine). 2000. *To err is human: Building a safer health system*. Washington, DC: National Academy Press.

IOM. 2001. *Crossing the quality chasm: A new health system for the 21st century*. Washington, DC: National Academy Press.

IPEC (Interprofessional Education Collaborative). 2011. *Core competencies for interprofessional collaborative practice: Report of an expert panel*. Washington, DC: IPEC.

McDonald, K. M., E. Schultz, L. Albin, N. Pineda, J. Lonhart, V. Sundaram, C. Smith-Spangler, J. Brustrom, E. Malcolm, L. Rohn, and S. Davies. 2014. *Care coordination measures atlas version 4* (Prepared by Stanford University under subcontract to American Institutes for Research on Contract No. HHSA290-2010-00005I). AHRQ Publication No. 14-0037-EF. Rockville, MD: Agency for Healthcare Research and Quality. http://www.ahrq.gov/professionals/prevention-chronic-care/improve/coordination/atlas2014 (accessed April 9, 2015).

MOH (Ministry of Health, Kingdom of Saudi Arabia). 2014. *The MOH, in collaboration with the Ministry of Education, evaluates the role of the health affairs directorates in educating on MERS CoronaVirus*. http://www.moh.gov.sa/en/Ministry/MediaCenter/News/Pages/News-2014-05-13-002.aspx (accessed March 17, 2015).

Moore, D. E., Jr., J. S. Green, and H. A. Gallis. 2009. Achieving desired results and improved outcomes: Integrating planning and assessment throughout learning activities. *Journal of Continuing Education in the Health Professions* 29(1):1-15.

National Center for Interprofessional Practice and Education. 2013. *Measurement instruments*. https://nexusipe.org/measurement-instruments (accessed April 9, 2015).

Nisbet, G., M. Lincoln, and S. Dunn. 2013. Informal interprofessional learning: An untapped opportunity for learning and change within the workplace. *Journal of Interprofessional Care* 27(6):469-475.

Oandasan, I., and S. Reeves. 2005. Key elements for interprofessional education. Part 1: The learner, the educator and the learning context. *Journal of Interprofessional Care* 19(Suppl. 1):21-38.

Olson, R., and A. Bialocerkowski. 2014. Interprofessional education in allied health: A systematic review. *Medical Education* 48(3):236-246.

Ovseiko, P. V., A. Heitmueller, P. Allen, S. M. Davies, G. Wells, G. A. Ford, A. Darzi, and A. M. Buchan. 2014. Improving accountability through alignment: The role of academic health science centres and networks in England. *BMC Health Services Research* 14:24.

Price, J. 2005. Complexity and interprofessional education. In *The theory-practice relationship in interprofessional education*, Ch. 8, edited by H. Colyer, M. Helme, and I. Jones. King's College, London: Higher Education Academy. Pp. 79-87.

Reeves, S., S. Lewin, S. Espin, and M. Zwarenstein. 2010. *Interprofessional teamwork for health and social care*. London: Wiley-Blackwell.

Reeves, S., J. Goldman, J. Gilbert, J. Tepper, I. Silver, E. Suter, and M. Zwarenstein. 2011. A scoping review to improve conceptual clarity of interprofessional interventions. *Journal of Interprofessional Care* 25(3):167-174.

Reeves, S., L. Perrier, J. Goldman, D. Freeth, and M. Zwarenstein. 2013. Interprofessional education: Effects on professional practice and healthcare outcomes (update). *Cochrane Database of Systematic Reviews* 3:CD002213.

Remington, T. L., M. A. Foulk, and B. C. Williams. 2006. Evaluation of evidence for interprofessional education. *The American Journal of Pharmaceutical Education* 70(3):66.

Ricketts, T. C., and E. P. Fraher. 2013. Reconfiguring health workforce policy so that education, training, and actual delivery of care are closely connected. *Health Affairs (Millwood)* 32(11):1874-1880.

Salas, E., and M. A. Rosen. 2013. Building high reliability teams: Progress and some reflections on teamwork training. *BMJ Quality and Safety* 22(5):369-373.

Salas, E., D. DiazGranados, C. Klein, C. S. Burke, K. C. Stagl, G. F. Goodwin, and S. M. Halpin. 2008a. Does team training improve team performance? A meta-analysis. *Human Factors: The Journal of the Human Factors and Ergonomics Society* 50(6):903-933.

Schmitz, C. C., and M. J. Cullen. 2015. *Evaluating interprofessional education and collaborative practice: What should I consider when selecting a measurement tool?* https://nexusipe.org/evaluating-ipecp (accessed April 9, 2015).

Thannhauser, J., S. Russell-Mayhew, and C. Scott. 2010. Measures of interprofessional education and collaboration. *Journal of Interprofessional Care* 24(4):336-349.

Valentine, M. A., I. M. Nembhard, and A. C. Edmondson. 2015. Measuring teamwork in health care settings: A review of survey instruments. *Medical Care* 53(4):e16-e30.

Walsh, K., S. Reeves, and S. Maloney. 2014. Exploring issues of cost and value in professional and interprofessional education. *Journal of Interprofessional Care* 28(6):493-494.

Weaver, L., A. McMurtry, J. Conklin, S. Brajtman, and P. Hall. 2011. Harnessing complexity science for interprofessional education development: A case study. *Journal of Research in Interprofessional Practice and Education* 2(1):100-120.

Weaver, S. J., M. A. Rosen, D. DiazGranados, E. H. Lazzara, R. Lyons, E. Salas, S. A. Knych, M. McKeever, L. Adler, M. Barker, and H. B. King. 2010. Does teamwork improve performance in the operating room? A multilevel evaluation. *Joint Commission Journal on Quality and Patient Safety* 36(3):133-142.

WHO (World Health Organization). 2010. *Framework for action on interprofessional education and collaborative practice*. Geneva: WHO.

WHO. 2011. *Transformative scale up of health professional education*. Geneva: WHO.

WHO. 2013. *Interprofessional collaborative practice in primary health care: Nursing and midwifery perspectives. Six case studies*. Geneva: WHO.

Zwarenstein, M., J. Goldman, and S. Reeves. 2009. Interprofessional collaboration: Effects of practice-based interventions on professional practice and healthcare outcomes. *Cochrane Database of Systematic Reviews* 3:CD000072.

1

Introduction

Global transformation is occurring at an unprecedented pace. Soaring population rates, climate change, rapid urbanization, technological innovation, and globalization all are intersecting in ways that would have been unthinkable just a few decades ago. Such convergences have dictated the critical need for improved communication and collaboration at both the global and local levels.

Within health and health care, new and different types of collaboration are emerging among and between the providers of health, welfare, and social care (Frenk et al., 2010). Interprofessional teamwork and collaborative practice are becoming key elements of efficient and productive efforts to promote health and treat patients. This work involves health and/or social professions that share a team or network identity and work closely together in an integrated and interdependent manner to solve problems, deliver services, and enhance health. Patients, families, consumers, and communities have traditionally been excluded as integral members of such collaborations despite repeated calls for their inclusion (Cox and Naylor, 2013; Hibbard, 2003; Hibbard et al., 2005; Hovey et al., 2011; IOM, 2003, 2006; WestRasmus et al., 2012; WHO, 2010). Yet, they are all part of the broader health system that according to Murray and Frenk (1999) is driven by three intrinsic goals: health, responsiveness, and fairness in financing—more specifically, improving the health of the population and enhancing the responsiveness of health systems to such important nonhealth dimensions as respect for patients and families, consumer satisfaction, and affordability of all households' contributions to the health system.

Effective interprofessional collaboration requires the alignment of values, skills, and resources toward attaining these goals (Cox and Naylor, 2013; Zwarenstein et al., 2009). In health care, this alignment not only results from a moral imperative to work together to combat a specific disease (e.g., cancer diagnosis and treatment) or public health crisis (e.g., the recent Ebola epidemic) but also increasingly, in western countries, is driven by concerns about the overall health of the population, the quality and safety of health care, and health care costs (IOM, 2000; Leonard et al., 2004; Nielsen et al., 2014; Reaves et al., 2014; Sands et al., 2008). Health care institutions around the world may have much to learn from sectors such as the airline industry that demonstrate effective implementation of teamwork for the purposes of minimizing errors and improving safety (Baker et al., 2006; de Korne et al., 2010; Helmreich et al., 1999; Manser, 2009; Shaw and Calder, 2008; WHO, 2009).

Inadequate preparation of health professionals for working together, especially in interprofessional teams, has been implicated in a range of adverse outcomes, including lower provider and patient satisfaction, greater numbers of medical errors and other patient safety issues, low workforce retention, system inefficiencies resulting in higher costs, and suboptimal community engagement (Epstein, 2014; IOM, 2003; WHO, 2010; Zwarenstein et al., 2009). But unlike other sectors—such as aviation, the military, and many for-profit corporations—that have been quick to integrate teamwork into their training, the health, welfare, and social care sectors often have been slower to implement team-based care and other models of collaboration, as well as the interprofessional education (IPE) that is necessary to support and improve collaboration (Baker et al., 2006; Miller et al., 2008; Salas and Rosen, 2013; Schmitt et al., 2011). This difference may be a reflection of differences in alignment. While the aviation industry closely aligns training, flying, and federal safety regulations, systems of education and health care delivery display little to no alignment. Other reasons also are believed to promote a reluctance to fully accept IPE, including a lack of systematic evidence for its effectiveness in improving health and system outcomes (e.g., Braithwaite and Travaglia, 2005; Reeves et al., 2013).

ORIGINS OF THE STUDY

In 2013, the Institute of Medicine's (IOM's) Global Forum on Innovation in Health Professional Education held two workshops on IPE. At these workshops, a number of questions were raised, the most important of which was, "What data and metrics are needed to evaluate the impact of IPE on individual, population, and system outcomes?" To answer this question, the Forum's individual sponsors (listed in Appendix D) requested that an IOM consensus committee be convened to examine the existing evidence on this complex issue and consider the potential design of future studies that could expand this evidence base. The committee's statement of task is presented in Box 1-1.

To fulfill the Forum's request, the committee employed a study process that included

- a balanced committee of experts vetted for biases and conflicts of interest;
- a commissioned paper (1) examining the best methods currently used for measuring the impact of IPE on collaborative practice, patient outcomes, or both, and (2) describing the challenges to conducting high-quality research linking IPE with measurable changes in patient and clinical practice outcomes (see Appendix A);
- an examination of recent review articles, conducted by three committee members using a format similar to that of the commissioned paper (see Appendix B);
- one day of open testimony from outside experts, which supplemented the knowledge of the committee members (see Appendix C for the agenda for this session);
- three days of closed-door deliberations during which the committee agreed upon its conclusions and recommendations; and
- virtual meetings during which the conclusions and recommendations presented in this report were finalized.

BOX 1-1
Statement of Task

An Institute of Medicine committee will examine the methods needed to measure the impact of interprofessional education (IPE) on collaborative practice, patient outcomes or both, as determined by the available evidence. Considerable research on IPE has focused on assessing student learning, but only recently have researchers begun looking beyond the classroom for impacts of IPE on such issues as patient safety, provider and patient satisfaction, quality of care, community health outcomes, and cost savings.

The committee will analyze the available data and information to determine the best methods for measuring the impact of IPE on specific aspects of health care delivery and health care systems functioning, such as IPE impacts on collaborative practice and patient outcomes (including safety and quality of care). Following review of the available evidence, the committee will recommend a range of different approaches based on the best available methodologies that measure the impact of IPE on collaborative practice, patient outcomes or both. The committee will also identify gaps where further research is needed. These recommendations will be targeted primarily at health professional educational leaders.

SCOPE AND ORGANIZATION OF THE REPORT

The committee identified a number of factors that complicate evaluation of the impact of IPE on patient, population, and system outcomes, but three factors dominated its deliberations and therefore receive particular attention in this report.

First, the context within which education interventions are implemented matters greatly (Barr et al., 2005; Thistlethwaite, 2012; see Appendix A). In the global context, most IPE studies are published in the English literature, with Canada, the United Kingdom, and the United States having the greatest presence, while developing countries have very few publications on the subject (Abu-Rish et al., 2012; Paradis and Reeves, 2013; Rodger and Hoffman, 2010; Sunguya et al., 2014). Drawing overarching conclusions is therefore difficult. Context likewise is important in examining the impact of education interventions from a national, community, or institutional perspective or even in comparing results from different points of care (clinical microsystems) within a single institution. The importance of context is especially salient given the rapid change that characterizes the health care system today.

Second, during the committee's open data gathering session (IOM, 2014), it was noted that although changes in interprofessional curricula are increasingly common and collaborative competencies are being written into accreditation standards, the outcomes of adopting these standards in a meaningful way remain unclear. It also was noted that the critical step in documenting the effectiveness of IPE across the education-to-practice continuum is better coordinating education interventions with ongoing health system redesign. The importance of context and the consequences of the lack of alignment between education reform and practice redesign in evaluating the outcomes of IPE are addressed in Chapter 2.

Third, it quickly became apparent that a common language and conceptual model are needed as a template for the design of education interventions and the analysis of IPE outcomes. During the committee's open session, the multiple and sometimes conflicting definitions with which the committee would have to grapple were highlighted, along with the wide variety of perspectives on how to define IPE and its outcomes and the lack of linearity and alignment of IPE; collaborative practice; and patient, population, and system outcomes (Cooper et al., 2004; Weaver et al., 2011). In short, there was support for a conceptual framework that could guide a common understanding of the impact of IPE (Clark, 2006; Reeves et al., 2011). Existing models for describing IPE and learning that the committee reviewed did not meet this need. Therefore, the committee created a comprehensive model that would allow for a description of IPE across the continuum of health professions education. The concepts and language developed for this model proved to be especially valuable in distinguishing between intermediate and more distal outcomes (i.e., between the acquisition of collaborative skills and the ultimate effects of IPE on individual, population, and system outcomes). This model is described in Chapter 3 and is referred to throughout Chapters 4 and 5.

The central goal of IPE is to produce a health workforce prepared to collaborate in new and different ways to yield positive impacts on the health of individuals, the communities in which they live, and the health systems that care for them (WHO, 2010). The need to strengthen the evidence base for linkages between IPE and these outcomes is described in Chapter 4. As a central focus of the report, Chapter 4 lays the foundation for the report's two recommendations provided in Chapter 4 and in Chapter 5, which call for the development of measures of collaborative performance that are effective across a broad range of learning environments and a mixed-methods approach to measuring the impact of IPE on individual, population, and system outcomes.

Chapter 4 relies heavily on the background paper commissioned by the committee to inform its deliberations (see Appendix A), as well as the committee-initiated synthesis of review articles on IPE published between 2010 and 2014 (see Appendix B). The conclusions and recommendations in Chapters 4 and 5 draw on the findings presented in these papers.

While the sponsors of this study are the primary audience for the report's conclusions and recommendations, other individuals and organizations that are responsible for funding education and health care delivery systems are intended audiences as well. This list would likely include accreditors of health professions education and those who provide resources for education reform and health system redesign, as well as government agencies that fund health professions education and university leadership associated with academic health centers. Individuals in these positions who are accountable for funding education and health systems would have particular responsibilities in this regard.

REFERENCES

Abu-Rish, E., S. Kim, L. Choe, L. Varpio, E. Malik, A. A. White, K. Craddick, K. Blondon, L. Robins, P. Nagasawa, A. Thigpen, L. L. Chen, J. Rich, and B. Zierler. 2012. Current trends in interprofessional education of health sciences students: A literature review. *Journal of Interprofessional Care* 26(6):444-451.

Baker, D. P., R. Day, and E. Salas. 2006. Teamwork as an essential component of high-reliability organizations. *Health Services Research* 41(4, pt. 2):1576-1598.

Barr, H., I. Koppel, S. Reeves, M. Hammick, and D. Freeth. 2005. *Effective interprofessional education: Assumption, argument and evidence.* Oxford and Malden: Blackwell Publishing.

Braithwaite, J., and J. F. Travaglia. 2005. *Inter-professional learning and clinical education: An overview of the literature*. Canberra, Australia: Braithwaite and Associates and the ACT (Australian Capital Territory) Health Department.

Clark, P. G. 2006. What would a theory of interprofessional education look like? Some suggestions for developing a theoretical framework for teamwork training. *Journal of Interprofessional Care* 20(6):577-589.

Cooper, H., S. Braye, and R. Geyer. 2004. Complexity and interprofessional education. *Learning in Health and Social Care* 3(4):179-189.

Cox, M., and M. Naylor. 2013. *Transforming patient care: Aligning interprofessional education with clinical practice redesign*. Proceedings of a Conference sponsored by the Josiah Macy Jr. Foundation in January 2013. New York: Josiah Macy Jr. Foundation. http://macyfoundation.org/docs/macy_pubs/JMF_TransformingPatientCare_Jan2013Conference_fin_Web.pdf (accessed March 17, 2014).

de Korne, D. F., J. D. van Wijngaarden, U. F. Hiddema, F. G. Bleeker, P. J. Pronovost, and N. S. Klazinga. 2010. Diffusing aviation innovations in a hospital in the Netherlands. *Joint Commission Journal on Quality and Patient Safety* 36(8):339-347.

Epstein, N. E. 2014. Multidisciplinary in-hospital teams improve patient outcomes: A review. *Surgical Neurology International* 5(Suppl 7):S295-S303.

Frenk, J., L. Chen, Z. A. Bhutta, J. Cohen, N. Crisp, T. Evans, H. Fineberg, P. Garcia, Y. Ke, P. Kelley, B. Kistnasamy, A. Meleis, D. Naylor, A. Pablos-Mendez, S. Reddy, S. Scrimshaw, J. Sepulveda, D. Serwadda, and H. Zurayk. 2010. Health professionals for a new century: Transforming education to strengthen health systems in an interdependent world. *Lancet* 376(9756):1923-1958.

Helmreich, R. L., A. C. Merritt, and J. A. Wilhelm. 1999. The evolution of crew resource management training in commercial aviation. *The International Journal of Aviation Psychology* 9(1):19-32.

Hibbard, J. H. 2003. Engaging health care consumers to improve the quality of care. *Medical Care* 41(1 Suppl):I61-I70.

Hibbard, J., E. Peters, P. Slovic, and M. Tusler. 2005. Can patients be part of the solution? Views on their role in preventing medical errors. *Medical Care Research and Review* 62(5):601-616.

Hovey, R., M. Dvorak, T. Burton, S. Worsham, J. Padilla, M. Hatlie, and A. Morck. 2011. Patient safety: A consumer's perspective. *Qualitative Health Research* 21(5):662-672.

IOM (Institute of Medicine). 2000. *To err is human: Building a safer health system*. Washington, DC: National Academy Press.

IOM. 2003. *Health professions education: A bridge to quality*. Washington, DC: The National Academies Press.

IOM. 2006. *Improving the quality of health care for mental and substance-use conditions*. Washington, DC: The National Academies Press.

IOM. 2014. *Open session for measuring the impact of interprofessional education (IPE) on collaborative practice and patient outcomes: A consensus study*. http://iom.national academies.org/Activities/Global/MeasuringtheImpactofInterprofessionalEducation/2014-OCT-07.aspx (accessed December 8, 2014).

Leonard, M., S. Graham, and D. Bonacum. 2004. The human factor: The critical importance of effective teamwork and communication in providing safe care. *Quality and Safety in Health Care* 13(Suppl. 1):i85-i90.

Manser, T. 2009. Teamwork and patient safety in dynamic domains of healthcare: A review of the literature. *Acta Anaesthesiologica Scandinavica* 53(2):143-151.

Miller, K. L., S. Reeves, M. Zwarenstein, J. D. Beales, C. Kenaszchuk, and L. G. Conn. 2008. Nursing emotion work and interprofessional collaboration in general internal medicine wards: A qualitative study. *Journal of Advanced Nursing* 64(4):332-343.

Murray, C. J. L., and J. A. Frenk. 1999. *WHO framework for health system performance assessment.* Global Programme on Evidence for Health Policy Discussion Paper No. 6. Geneva: WHO.

Nielsen, M., J. N. Olayiwola, P. Grundy, and K. Grumbach. 2014. *The patient-centered medical home's impact on cost & quality: An annual update of the evidence, 2012-2013.* Washington, DC: Patient-Centered Primary Care Collaborative.

Paradis, E., and S. Reeves. 2013. Key trends in interprofessional research: A macrosociological analysis from 1970 to 2010. *Journal of Interprofessional Care* 27(2):113-122.

Reaves, E. J., A. M. Arwady, L. G. Mabande, D. A. Thoroughman, and J. M. Montgomery. 2014. Control of Ebola virus disease—Firestone district, Liberia, 2014. *Morbidity and Mortality Weekly Report* 63(42):959-965.

Reeves, S., J. Goldman, J. Gilbert, J. Tepper, I. Silver, E. Suter, and M. Zwarenstein. 2011. A scoping review to improve conceptual clarity of interprofessional interventions. *Journal of Interprofessional Care* 25(3):167-174.

Reeves, S., L. Perrier, J. Goldman, D. Freeth, and M. Zwarenstein. 2013. Interprofessional education: Effects on professional practice and healthcare outcomes (update). *Cochrane Database of Systematic Reviews* 3:CD002213.

Rodger, S., and S. Hoffman. 2010. Where in the world is interprofessional education? A global environmental scan. *Journal of Interprofessional Care* 24(5):479-491.

Salas, E., and M. A. Rosen. 2013. Building high reliability teams: Progress and some reflections on teamwork training. *BMJ Quality and Safety* 22(5):369-373.

Sands, S. A., P. Stanley, and R. Charon. 2008. Pediatric narrative oncology: Interprofessional training to promote empathy, build teams, and prevent burnout. *Journal of Supportive Oncology* 6(7):307-312.

Schmitt, M. H., D. C. J. Baldwin, and S. Reeves. 2011. Continuing interprofessional education: Collaborative learning for collaborative practice. In *Continuing medical education: Looking back, planning ahead,* edited by D. K. Wentz. Hanover, NH: Dartmouth College Press. Pp. 300-316.

Shaw, J., and K. Calder. 2008. Aviation is not the only industry: Healthcare could look wider for lessons on patient safety. *Quality and Safety in Health Care* 17(5):314.

Sunguya, B. F., M. Jimba, J. Yasuoka, and W. Hinthong. 2014. Interprofessional education for whom?: Challenges and lessons learned from its implementation in developed countries and their application to developing countries: A systematic review. *PLoS ONE* 9(5):e96724.

Thistlethwaite, J. 2012. Interprofessional education: A review of context, learning and the research agenda. *Medical Education* 46(1):58-70.

Weaver, L., A. McMurtry, J. Conklin, S. Brajtman, and P. Hall. 2011. Harnessing complexity science for interprofessional education development: A case study. *Journal of Research in Interprofessional Practice and Education* 2(1):100-120.

WestRasmus, E. K., F. Pineda-Reyes, M. Tamez, and J. M. Westfall. 2012. Promotores de salud and community health workers: An annotated bibliography. *Family Community Health* 35(2):172-182.

WHO (World Health Organization). 2009. *Better knowledge for safer care: Human factors in patient safety review of topics and tools. Report for methods and measures working group of WHO patient safety.* Geneva: WHO.

WHO. 2010. *Framework for action on interprofessional education and collaborative practice.* Geneva: WHO.

Zwarenstein, M., J. Goldman, and S. Reeves. 2009. Interprofessional collaboration: Effects of practice-based interventions on professional practice and healthcare outcomes. *Cochrane Database of Systematic Reviews* 3:CD000072.

2

Alignment of Education and Health Care Delivery Systems

A critical factor in examining the effectiveness of interprofessional education (IPE) is the context in which the education intervention is implemented. National, institutional, and point-of-care differences impact study design and analysis and complicate comparisons across studies (as discussed in more detail in Chapter 4). What may be less well appreciated is that context also is a critical factor in determining whether education initiatives in general and IPE interventions in particular are effective and worthy of investment.

THE NEED FOR GREATER ALIGNMENT

Coordinated planning among educators, health system leaders, and policy makers is a prerequisite for creating an optimal learning environment and an effective health workforce (Cox and Naylor, 2013). Coordinated planning requires that educators be cognizant of health systems' ongoing redesign efforts, and that health system leaders recognize the realities of educating and training a competent health workforce. Further, education and health systems are impacted separately or together by a wide variety of policies, necessitating joint planning among educators, policy makers, and workforce leaders. This is especially important when health systems are undergoing rapid changes, as they are across much of the world today (Coker et al., 2008). The One Health movement may offer strategies for bridging potential policy, education, and workforce divides in a complex environment given that emerging zoonotic and environmental threats to human health require a multisector, coordinated response that aligns activities, strategies, policies, and funding (One Health Initiative, n.d.; WHO, n.d.).

Despite calls for greater alignment, however, education reform is rarely well integrated with health system redesign (Cox and Naylor, 2013; Earnest and Brandt, 2014; Frenk et al., 2010; Ricketts and Fraher, 2013; WHO, 2010, 2011). Accountability for workforce and health outcomes often is dispersed between academic health centers and health care networks (Ovseiko et al., 2014). Possible exceptions include the rare cases in which ministries of education and health work together on individual initiatives (Booth, 2014; Frenk et al., 2010; MOH, 2014). Even when the education and practice communities work together, however, collaboration tends to be restricted to a single health profession.

> "Education reform is rarely well integrated with health system redesign."

In the United States, several federal and state team-based health system redesign initiatives are currently under way, such as Vermont Blueprint for Health, the Center for Medicare & Medicaid Innovation (CMMI), and the Veterans Health Administration's (VHA's) patient-centered medical homes (CMMI, n.d.; Department of Vermont Health Access, 2014; Klein, 2011). Yet as with many other IPE developments around the globe, such as those in Australia, Germany, Japan, and the United Kingdom, these initiatives display no systematic linkages between the education and practice communities in their design and implementation and demonstrate very few explicit efforts to support and learn about IPE. One exception in the United States is the VHA health system, where Centers of Excellence in Primary Care Education have been established as an integral part of an enterprise-wide effort to redesign the VHA's primary care delivery system by integrating purposeful IPE with team-based care (Gilman et al., 2014; Rugen et al., 2014; VA, 2015).

Despite isolated efforts to the contrary, the separation of governance and accountability for education and patient care is the rule for many countries around the world. In the United States, for example, although some deans of schools of medicine are involved in health system oversight, this generally is not the case for the academic leaders of other health professional schools within and across institutions of higher education. This makes joint planning for linking IPE to practice more difficult, particularly for the vast majority of health professional schools that are not housed in academic health centers.

Bringing together academic leaders alone also has significant limitations, as evidenced by the work of Batalden and Davidoff (2007) on quality improvement. Batalden and Davidoff define quality improvement as "the combined and unceasing efforts of everyone—healthcare professionals, patients and their families, researchers, payers, planners and educators—to make the changes that will lead to better patient outcomes (health), better system performance (care) and better professional development (learning)" (p. 2). In keeping with this definition, alignment is needed between the entities responsible and accountable for educating the health workforce and delivering care if IPE is to have beneficial effects on health and health care systems.

Community-based health initiatives have the potential to enable better alignment of IPE and health care delivery. In British Columbia, for example, Jarvis-Selinger and colleagues (2008) examined university–community collaborations for interprofessional development through work with Aboriginal communities. The authors note that "interprofessional approaches to education and community practice have the potential to contribute to improvements in access to care, as well as health professional recruitment in underserved communities" (p. 61).

Student-run clinics, interprofessional training wards, and other service-learning initiatives are other venues in which interprofessional teamwork can flourish in tandem with community-based practice (e.g., Haggarty and Dalcin, 2014; Holmqvist et al., 2012). However, these initiatives generally are voluntary, do not purposefully pursue IPE or faculty development for interprofessional collaborative practice, and lack sufficient human and financial resources for conducting robust evaluations (Holmqvist et al., 2012; Khorasani et al., 2010; Meah et al., 2009; Society of Student-Run Free Clinics, 2011).

CONCLUSION

Aligning the organizations responsible for IPE and collaborative practice will allow for more robust evaluations of IPE interventions and will facilitate the creation of feedback loops between practice and education.

Conclusion 1. Without a purposeful and more comprehensive system of engagement between the education and health care delivery systems, evaluating the impact of IPE interventions on health and system outcomes will be difficult.

Such alignment will necessarily involve the active participation of education leadership (in public and private universities and their health professional schools), health care delivery system leadership (in teaching health systems, centers, and clinics), health professions societies, and public health authorities. It also will require the assumption of joint accountability for both patient and community health, and shared adoption of competency-driven approaches to instructional design and evaluation of health and system outcomes.

Better alignment will necessitate that regulators, accreditors, and other professional bodies strengthen collaborative partnerships between health professions education programs and health systems in support of interprofessional learning by requiring the adoption of competency-based expectations for accreditation. At the same time, those who provide resources for system redesign, innovative practice models, and maintenance of the overall health system can facilitate progress by offering economic incentives for better alignment.

Achieving greater alignment entails significant challenges resulting from the complexity of the relationships among the various stakeholders and their sometimes overlapping responsibilities. Examples of this complexity include the joint responsibility for IPE of universities, affiliated clinical training sites, and health system employers across the continuum of education and practice; the divided responsibility of professional and governmental health professions regulatory bodies; and the overlapping roles of local, regional, national, and international policy makers. Given this complexity, the concept of alignment may best be regarded as having both vertical and horizontal dimensions, each composed of continuously interacting systems designed to achieve (but not always achieving) improved efficiency and effectiveness.

The overall result of this complexity is that although the logic of alignment between education and practice is widely accepted, it has been slow to take hold (Chen et al., 2015; Cox and Naylor, 2013; Earnest and Brandt, 2014; Frenk et al., 2010; Ricketts and Fraher, 2013; WHO, 2010, 2011). Engagement around the importance of alignment would be greatly accelerated by evidence from demonstration projects convincingly linking IPE (and other education interventions) to positive outcomes. Creating a more conducive environment for such engagement will require strong advocacy and leadership, well-targeted policy changes, and innovative incentives.

Such a strategy could be guided by the many examples around the world of effective relationships among universities, government, and industry (Martin, 2000; Ovseiko et al., 2014). Strategies specific to IPE were the subject of a recent conference (Cox and Naylor, 2013). Among the many recommendations made by participants in that conference were including patients and communities in advocacy initiatives, changing professional and hospital accreditation standards to explicitly promote team-based care, creating new models of resource sharing between education and health care institutions, and demonstrating a positive value proposition for linking IPE and collaborative practice. Giving the public a direct voice in health professions governance (for example, by including patients and representatives of consumer organizations on boards of directors), creating joint accreditation standards and joint accreditation boards (Joint Accreditation, 2013), and using financial incentives to promote change in health professions education and health care delivery may be especially powerful.[1]

REFERENCES

Batalden, P. B., and F. Davidoff. 2007. What is "quality improvement" and how can it transform healthcare? *Quality & Safety in Health Care* 16(1):2-3.

Booth, D. 2014. *Remarks by U.S. Ambassador Donald Booth at the inauguration of the new medical education initiative Ambo University.* http://ethiopia.usembassy.gov/latest_embassy_news/remarks/remarks-by-u.s.-ambassador-donald-booth-on-inauguration-of-the-new-medical-education-initiative-ambo-university (accessed January 12, 2015).

Chen, F., C. C. Delnat, and D. Gardner. 2015. The current state of academic centers for interprofessional education. *Journal of Interprofessional Care* 14:1-2.

CMMI (Center for Medicare & Medicaid Innovation). n.d. *The CMS Innovation Center.* http://innovation.cms.gov (accessed January 28, 2015).

Coker, R., R. A. Atun, and M. McKee. 2008. *Health systems and the challenge of communicable diseases: Experiences from Europe and Latin America, European Observatory on Health Systems and Policies Series.* Maidenhead and New York: McGraw-Hill Education.

Cox, M., and M. Naylor. 2013. *Transforming patient care: Aligning interprofessional education with clinical practice redesign.* Proceedings of a Conference sponsored by the Josiah Macy Jr. Foundation in January 2013. New York: Josiah Macy Jr. Foundation. http://macyfoundation.org/docs/macy_pubs/JMF_TransformingPatientCare_Jan2013Conference_fin_Web.pdf (accessed March 17, 2014).

Department of Vermont Health Access. 2014. *Vermont Blueprint for health: 2013 annual report (January 30, 2014).* Williston, VT: Department of Vermont Health Access.

Earnest, M., and B. Brandt. 2014. Aligning practice redesign and interprofessional education to advance triple aim outcomes. *Journal of Interprofessional Care* 28(6):497-500.

Frenk, J., L. Chen, Z. A. Bhutta, J. Cohen, N. Crisp, T. Evans, H. Fineberg, P. Garcia, Y. Ke, P. Kelley, B. Kistnasamy, A. Meleis, D. Naylor, A. Pablos-Mendez, S. Reddy, S. Scrimshaw, J. Sepulveda, D. Serwadda, and H. Zurayk. 2010. Health professionals for a new century: Transforming education to strengthen health systems in an interdependent world. *Lancet* 376(9756):1923-1958.

Gilman, S. C., D. A. Chokshi, J. L. Bowen, K. W. Rugen, and M. Cox. 2014. Connecting the dots: Interprofessional health education and delivery system redesign at the veterans health administration. *Academic Medicine* 89(8):1113-1116.

Haggarty, D., and D. Dalcin. 2014. Student-run clinics in Canada: An innovative method of delivering interprofessional education. *Journal of Interprofessional Care* 28(6):570-572.

Holmqvist, M., C. Courtney, R. Meili, and A. Dick. 2012. Student-run clinics: Opportunities for interprofessional education and increasing social accountability. *Journal of Research in Interprofessional Practice and Education* 2(3):264-277.

IOM (Institute of Medicine). 2014. *Graduate medical education that meets the nation's health needs.* Washington, DC: The National Academies Press.

Jarvis-Selinger, S., K. Ho, H. N. Lauscher, Y. Liman, E. Stacy, R. Woollard, and D. Buote. 2008. Social accountability in action: University-community collaboration in the development of an interprofessional aboriginal health elective. *Journal of Interprofessional Care* 22(Suppl. 1):61-72.

---

[1] Using financial incentives to promote clinical workforce reform is one of the themes of a 2014 Institute of Medicine report (IOM, 2014).

Joint Accreditation. 2013. *Joint Accreditation for interprofessional education. Medicine, pharmacy and nursing.* http://www.jointaccreditation.org (accessed March 17, 2015).

Khorasani, S., T. Berg, M. Khorasani, and S. Kolker. 2010. An innovative model for interprofessional education and practice: A student-run interprofessional rehabilitation medicine clinic. *University of British Columbia Medical Journal* 2(1):39-42.

Klein, S. 2011. The Veterans Health Administration: Implementing patient-centered medical homes in the nation's largest integrated delivery system. *Commonwealth Fund* 16(1537): 1-24.

Martin, M. 2000. *Managing university-industry relations: A study of institutional practices from 12 different countries.* http://unesdoc.unesco.org/images/0012/001202/120290e.pdf (accessed March 17, 2015).

Meah, Y. S., E. L. Smith, and D. C. Thomas. 2009. Student-run health clinic: Novel arena to educate medical students on systems-based practice. *Mount Sinai Journal of Medicine* 76(4):344-356.

MOH (Ministry of Health, Kingdom of Saudi Arabia). 2014. *The MOH, in collaboration with the Ministry of Education, evaluates the role of the health affairs directorates in educating on MERS CoronaVirus.* http://www.moh.gov.sa/en/Ministry/MediaCenter/News/Pages/News-2014-05-13-002.aspx (accessed March 17, 2015).

One Health Initiative. n.d. *One Health Initiative will unite human and veterinary medicine.* http://www.onehealthinitiative.com (accessed March 17, 2015).

Ovseiko, P. V., A. Heitmueller, P. Allen, S. M. Davies, G. Wells, G. A. Ford, A. Darzi, and A. M. Buchan. 2014. Improving accountability through alignment: The role of academic health science centres and networks in England. *BMC Health Services Research* 14:24.

Ricketts, T. C., and E. P. Fraher. 2013. Reconfiguring health workforce policy so that education, training, and actual delivery of care are closely connected. *Health Affairs (Millwood)* 32(11):1874-1880.

Rugen, K. W., S. A. Watts, S. L. Janson, L. A. Angelo, M. Nash, S. A. Zapatka, R. Brienza, S. C. Gilman, J. L. Bowen, and J. M. Saxe. 2014. Veteran affairs centers of excellence in primary care education: Transforming nurse practitioner education. *Nursing Outlook* 62(2):78-88.

Society of Student-Run Free Clinics. 2011. *Presentation abstracts.* 2011 International Conference: Student-Run Clinics Across the Continuum of Care, January 21, 2011. Houston, TX: Society of Student-Run Free Clinics.

VA (U.S. Department of Veterans Affairs). 2015. *Office of Academic Affiliations: VA Centers of Excellence in Primary Care Education (CoEPCE).* http://www.va.gov/OAA/coepce (accessed March 17, 2015).

WHO (World Health Organization). 2010. *Framework for action on interprofessional education and collaborative practice.* Geneva: WHO.

WHO. 2011. *Transformative scale up of health professional education.* Geneva: WHO.

WHO. n.d. *Managing zoonotic public health risks at the human–animal–ecosystem interface.* Geneva: WHO.

3

Conceptual Framework for Measuring the Impact of IPE

To date, the interprofessional education (IPE) literature has generally focused on formal and intentionally planned education and training programs (Freeth et al., 2005a,b; Nisbet et al., 2013). Most models of IPE have emphasized the characteristics of educational activities (e.g., type and duration of exposure) and learning outcomes. Some have addressed when IPE should occur (e.g., before or after licensure or certification) (Reeves et al., 2011). Fewer have explicitly considered where IPE occurs (e.g., classroom, clinical practice, or community settings) or what type of learning is most suited to a particular environment (D'Amour and Oandasan, 2004; Purden, 2005). Fewer still have examined patient, population, or system outcomes (Reeves et al., 2011, 2013).

One model reviewed by the committee links a number of concepts related to IPE (see Figure 3-1) (Owen and Schmitt, 2013). This model builds on earlier thinking about a patient-centered approach to learning in the health professions and describes the intersections of IPE with basic education, graduate education, and continuing IPE; it also captures the understanding that point-of-care learning is a key component of lifelong learning (Josiah Macy Jr. Foundation, 2010). This broad definition of continuing education encompasses all learning (formal, informal, workplace, serendipitous) that enhances understanding and improves patient care (IOM, 2010; Nisbet et al., 2013). All of these elements are important in linking IPE to individual, population, and system outcomes.

This model became the basis for the committee's consideration of more complex concepts than those generally used in designing IPE, understanding the role and utility of informal learning, and evaluating the outcomes of

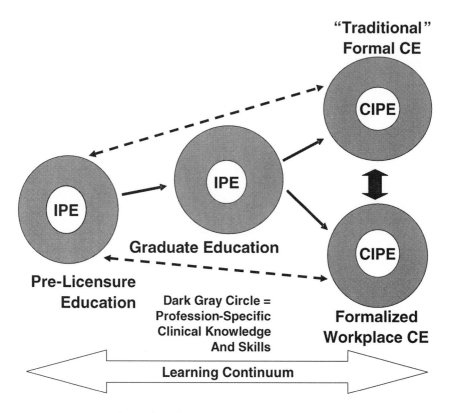

FIGURE 3-1 An enhanced professional education model capturing essential concepts of interprofessional education.
NOTE: CE = continuing education; CIPE = continuing interprofessional education; IPE = interprofessional education.
SOURCE: Owen and Schmitt, 2013.
© 2013 The Alliance for Continuing Education in the Health Professions, the Society for Academic Continuing Medical Education, and the Council on Continuing Medical Education, Association for Hospital Medical Education. Published online in Wiley Online Library (wileyonlinelibrary.com). doi: 10.1002/chp.21173.

both formal and informal types of IPE. These concepts include the developmental stages of a professional's career across the learning continuum, the incorporation of IPE into formal professional education across the developmental stages of a career, and the distinction between traditional formal continuing education (e.g., "update" models) and planned or serendipitous workplace learning (Lloyd et al., 2014; Nowlen, 1988). In addition, identifying the many activities that drive the need for effective evaluation of collaborative patient-centered practice is viewed as important by a number of groups and individuals (Baldwin et al., 2010; IPEC, 2011; Schmitt et al., 2011). These activities include those focused on patient safety, quality improvement, and team-based care, as well as population health and cost considerations. To date, these concepts have not been explicitly delineated in a comprehensive, well-conceived model of IPE.

The importance of context and the role of informal learning have been acknowledged by many authors (Eraut, 2004; Freeth et al., 2005a). In the United States, for example, leaders of U.S. health care systems (Fihn et al., 2014; Jones and Lunge, 2014; Department of Vermont Health Access, 2014) describe efforts to create teams, engage new types of workers, implement quality improvement, and collect population data in their health systems. In these efforts, a variety of positive outcomes have resulted from the deployment of new interprofessional models of care that stress the value of workplace learning rather than formal educational activities. These large-scale system redesign efforts underline the importance of incorporating what has been called the untapped opportunity for learning and change within practice environments offered by workplace learning, individual and organizational performance improvement efforts, and patient safety programs (Nisbet et al., 2013). However, participants in such transformative initiatives do not always recognize informal activities as "learning" when those activities are part of everyday practice (Eraut, 2004). Moreover, education and health system leaders may fail to consider the possibility of using workplace learning at earlier stages of the education continuum.

The need for better alignment between education and health systems and across the various phases of the education continuum is reinforced by large-scale transformative efforts. Without purposeful alignment, there is no feedback loop between education and practice or across the education continuum itself, and informal activities are not recognized or maximized as learning for everyone involved (students, health professionals, patients, families, and others). Too often students are directed to the classroom for their formal or foundational learning and only later to practice environments for short periods of time for application of those concepts, without a structured approach for learning in different environments.

> "Too often students are directed to the classroom for their formal or foundational learning and only later to practice environments for short periods of time for application of those concepts, without a structured approach for learning in different environments."

AN INTERPROFESSIONAL MODEL OF CONTINUOUS LEARNING

Following an extensive literature search for interprofessional models of learning, the committee determined that no existing models sufficiently incorporate all of the components needed to guide future studies. As a result, the committee developed a conceptual model that encompasses the education-to-practice continuum; a broad array of learning, health, and system outcomes; and major enabling and interfering factors. The committee puts forth this model with the understanding that it will need to be tested empirically and may need to be adapted to the particular settings in which it is applied. For example, educational structures and terminology differ considerably around the world, and the model may need to be modified to suit local or national conditions. However, the model's overarching concepts—a learning continuum; learning-, health-, and system-related outcomes; and major enabling and interfering factors—would remain.

Enabling and interfering factors can impact outcomes and influence program evaluation directly or indirectly. Diverse payment structures and differences in professional and organizational cultures generate obstacles to effective interprofessional work and evaluation, while positive changes in workforce and financing policies may enable more effective collaboration and foster robust interprofessional evaluation.

An Interprofessional Conceptual Model for Evaluating Outcomes

The interprofessional learning continuum (IPLC) model shown in Figure 3-2 encompasses four interrelated components: a learning continuum; the outcomes of learning; individual and population health outcomes; system outcomes such as organizational changes, system efficiencies, and cost-effectiveness; and the major enabling and interfering factors that influence implementation and overall outcomes. It must be emphasized that successful application of this model is dependent on how well the interdependent education and health care systems, as described in the previous chapter, are aligned.

This model illustrates the developmental and ongoing nature of organized (formal) IPE and workplace (informal) learning that occur as health professionals prepare for practice and progress throughout their careers. IPE is an all-encompassing term for both formal and informal learning interventions across the education-to-practice continuum; however, the model also distinguishes among the different stages and types of professional development (foundational education, graduate education, and continuing professional development) (Reeves et al., 2011), as well as the ideally increasing percentage of overall IPE that occurs across these stages.

IPE activities generally comprise a small fraction of overall educational

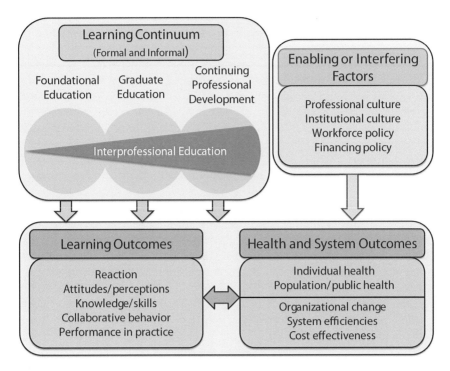

FIGURE 3-2 The interprofessional learning continuum (IPLC) model.
NOTE: For this model, "graduate education" encompasses any advanced formal or supervised health professions training taking place between completion of foundational education and entry into unsupervised practice.

activities early in the learning continuum, when students are being immersed in the values and information of their chosen profession and when the formation of professional identity is critical (Buring et al., 2009; Wagner and Reeves, 2015). As learning shifts from the classroom to the practice or community environment, interprofessional work takes on greater significance. Learning becomes more relationship based and involves increasingly more complex interactions with others, including patients, families, and communities. While the model does not visually display the integral role these individuals and groups play, they increasingly are emerging as important members of the collaborative team.

IPE may be formal or informal at any point across the education-to-practice continuum, but informal learning (planned or serendipitous workplace learning) increases as students progress in their education and as graduates become fully licensed and certified practitioners. This is one area in which local or national adaptation of the model would be necessary. Although the vast majority of health professionals are licensed and/or certi-fied to practice, for example, there are emerging professions and individual country health workforce circumstances that would necessitate ongoing adjustments to the model. Some health professions are not licensed because licensure is not required for employment. Other emerging professions, such as integrated health and health coaching, have certification requirements, while health educators and social service workers have variable require-ments depending on where the work is taking place (Healthcare Workforce Partnership of Western Mass, n.d.; SocialWorkLicensure.org, 2015; U.S. Department of Labor Bureau of Labor Statistics, 2014). By incorporating individual adaptations, the model allows for mapping the specific charac-teristics of an IPE intervention—timing, setting, and approach—to inter-mediate learning outcomes, and these, in turn, to specific types of health and system outcomes (Goldman et al., 2009; Oandasan and Reeves, 2005; Reeves et al., 2011). The model also takes into account the key factors (context, culture, and policy) that strongly influence, and in many cases confound, the design and analysis of any education intervention. Again, specific enabling and interfering factors will vary by setting and country. Specific health and system outcomes may also differ based on location and may include additional key indicators of health system performance, such as access to care and quality of care, possibly as they relate to the social determinants of health.

Furthermore, the model emphasizes that formal curricular interven-tions need to be designed intentionally to align specific interprofessional competencies with the professional's developmental stage (Dow et al., 2014; Wagner and Reeves, 2015). Some refer to this as the "treatment and dose" of IPE, denoting what the intervention should be and how much of it is needed to produce a measurable learning outcome. Whether an interven-tion leads to a measurable health or system outcome will likely depend on the interplay of multiple factors with particular confounding influences (see Chapter 4 for more detailed discussion of this topic).

Education and Training Pathways

The required education and training pathways for health professionals vary greatly in length, complexity, and sequencing and can differ within professions around the world. But in many places and for most health professions, formal education is highly regulated by accreditation, while informal workplace learning is influenced by the practice environment, including certification and licensing standards that are specific to each profession. In the committee's model, these concepts are incorporated in the three core developmental stages for health professionals: foundational education, graduate education, and continuing professional development (both formal and informal).

Foundational education is the educational entry point to a profession. Learners are novices who are provided basic content foundational to their profession. With the introduction of core competencies for interprofessional collaborative practice and new accreditation standards, IPE increasingly is being introduced at this early stage (CIHC, 2010; Curtin University, 2011; IPEC, 2011) and has been shown to have positive learning outcomes (Barr et al., 2005; Hawkes et al., 2013; Nisbet et al., 2008). Organized, formal IPE activities provide the basic underpinnings of collaborative competence. They generally are didactic or simulated or occur in highly supervised clinical environments.

For some professions, additional preparation is required in the form of graduate education or specialty training that is characterized by growing levels of independence. During this stage, supervisors or preceptors provide more complex situational learning experiences, while supervision for less complex situations decreases. Required competencies at this stage increasingly incorporate interprofessional practice skills such as practice-based learning and improvement and system-based practice (ACGME, 2013).

As health systems become more complex, there is increasing impetus to incorporate continuous improvement strategies so the system can evolve into a "learning organization" (deBurca, 2000; IOM, 2010). Accordingly, traditional approaches to continuing health professions education are moving beyond updating an individual professional's knowledge or skills in an area of specialization toward competency development and performance improvement in practice, including interprofessional collaborative practice skills in integrated systems of care and in community settings (ABMS, 2015; Cervero and Gaines, 2014). Increasingly, models for health professions competence and performance link learning to organizational outcomes, including patient and population benefits (e.g., improved individual and community health and system efficiencies such as cost reduction) (Davis et al., 1999; Forsetlund et al., 2009; Moore et al., 2009; WHO, 2010).

This shift in focus is fueling renewed interest in the role of workplace learning as part of everyday practice in the continuing professional development stage of a health professional's career (Gilman et al., 2014; Josiah Macy Jr. Foundation, 2010; Kitto et al., 2014; Marsick and Volpe, 1999; Regehr and Mylopoulos, 2008; Teunissen and Dornan, 2008). Nisbet and colleagues (2013, p. 469) propose a concept involving various types of workplace learning ranging from "the implicit unplanned learning . . . to more deliberative explicit focus on learning, where learning occurs through and is a central part of everyday work practice." This notion encompasses formal continuing education activities for maintaining licensure or certification as well as interprofessional development activities for informal on-the-job learning.

Charting Expectations for Interprofessional Learning

Against the backdrop of educational stages that guide IPE programming and evaluation, the planning for learner competency and performance benefits from charting developmental expectations for mastery of competencies, including interprofessional skills linked to particular learning outcomes (Dow et al., 2014; Wagner and Reeves, 2015). Charting expectations for individual learners along the learning continuum provides markers for planning, implementing, and evaluating IPE activities at appropriate times and intervals that align with the educational path of other learners, and establishes the basis for a progression of learner assessments.

As used by some health professions, the concepts of expectations, competencies, and entrustable professional activities are outcome markers (e.g., knowledge, skills, attitudes, behavior) that can be achieved progressively along the continuum of a learner's professional development (Mulder et al., 2010; ten Cate, 2013). These concepts take the learner from the earliest point of education and training through graduation and on to unsupervised practice. Assessment should be ongoing and feedback continuous to ensure that students achieve and demonstrate the competencies needed to move on to the next level of learning and development. Such an approach also can have value in resource-poor settings provided the educational design is adapted to address local health needs (Gruppen et al., 2012).

Levels of Learner Outcomes for Impact

Donald Kirkpatrick's (1959, 1967, 1994) training evaluation model has frequently been referenced as a model for the evaluation of formal IPE interventions (e.g., Gillan et al., 2011; Grymonpre et al., 2010; Hammick et al., 2007; Robben et al., 2012; Theilen et al., 2013). Kirkpatrick's four levels of outcomes—reaction, learning, behavior, and results—have been adapted by others (Weaver and Rosen, 2013), but the expansions of Barr et al. (2005) and Hammick et al. (2007) to include additional levels is increasingly being used in IPE (Mosley et al., 2012; Reeves et al., 2015) (see Table 3-1).

While the typology in Table 3-1 has provided a useful way of categorizing possible outcomes linked to IPE, the committee found it helpful to look back to Kirkpatrick's original model and its intent in developing the new interprofessional learning model depicted in Figure 3-2. For Kirkpatrick (1959), as well as Miller (1990), the highest form of learning outcome is *performance in practice* on a daily basis in complex systems—a learned ability linked to formal training or the development of expertise over time. While the model retains its focus on most of the learning outcomes in Table 3-1 (reaction, changes in attitudes/perceptions, changes in collabora-

TABLE 3-1 Kirkpatrick's Expanded Outcomes Typology

Level 1: Learner's reaction	Learners' views on the learning experience and its interprofessional nature
Level 2a: Modification of attitudes/perceptions	Changes in reciprocal attitudes or perceptions between participant groups; changes in attitudes or perceptions regarding the value and/or use of team approaches to caring for a specific client group
Level 2b: Acquisition of knowledge/skills	Including knowledge and skills linked to interprofessional collaboration
Level 3: Behavioral change	Individuals' transfer of interprofessional learning to their practice setting and their changed professional practice
Level 4a: Change in organizational practice	Wider changes in the organization and delivery of care
Level 4b: Benefits to patients, families, and communities	Improvements in health or well-being of patients, families, and communities

SOURCE: Adapted from Reeves et al., 2015. For more information, visit http://tandfonline.com/loi/ijic.

tive behavior), it reinstates the outcome of performance in practice. In the model, performance is seen as an outcome beyond collaborative behavior, focused on working in complex systems using a complex set of skills to potentially impact changes in health care delivery (see Figure 3-2).

Use of the Kirkpatrick model has been questioned by some who argue that it was not originally designed to look at complex organizational or consumer change (Bates, 2004; Yardley and Dornan, 2012). In recognition of this complexity, the committee decided to differentiate (intermediate) learning outcomes from (final) health and system outcomes. In doing so, the committee incorporated a range of health outcomes (individual health, population/public health) and system outcomes (organizational change, systems efficiencies, cost-effectiveness) to show the possible (final) impact of IPE.

CONCLUSION

Having a comprehensive conceptual model provides a taxonomy and framework for discussion of the evidence linking IPE with learning, health, and system outcomes. Without such a model, evaluating the impact of IPE on the health of patients and populations and on health system structure and function is difficult and perhaps impossible.

The committee's proposed model (see Figure 3-2) is the type of model needed to highlight desired system outcomes, such as those noted in Chapter 1 (health, responsiveness, and fairness in financing), that can be attributed to IPE. While this particular model requires empirical testing, the further development and widespread adoption of this type of model could be driven by professional organizations with a stake in promoting, overseeing, and evaluating IPE. Its adoption would require the active participation of the broader education, regulatory, and research communities, as well as of health care delivery system leaders and policy makers.

In sum, adoption of a conceptual model of IPE could focus related research and evaluation on individual, population, and system outcomes that go beyond learning and testing of team function. By visualizing the entire IPE process, such a model illuminates the different environments where IPE occurs, as well as the importance of aligning education and practice, enabling more systemic and robust research. Wider adoption of a model of this type could bring greater uniformity to the design of IPE studies and allow consideration of the entire IPE process within its very complex environment.

Conclusion 2. Having a comprehensive conceptual model would greatly enhance the description and purpose of IPE interventions and their potential impact. Such a model would provide a consistent taxonomy and framework for strengthening the evidence base linking IPE with health and system outcomes.

REFERENCES

ABMS (American Board of Medical Specialties). 2015. *Promoting CPD through MOC.* http://www.abms.org/initiatives/committing-to-physician-quality-improvement/promoting-cpd-through-moc (accessed March 17, 2015).

ACGME (Accreditation Council for Graduate Medical Education). 2013. *ACGME program requirements for graduate medical education in internal medicine.* https://www.acgme.org/acgmeweb/Portals/0/PFAssets/2013-PR-FAQ-PIF/140_internal_medicine_07012013.pdf (accessed December 29, 2014).

Baldwin, M., J. Hashima, J. M. Guise, W. T. Gregory, A. Edelman, and S. Segel. 2010. Patient-centered collaborative care: The impact of a new approach to postpartum rounds on residents' perception of their work environment. *Journal of Graduate Medical Education* 2(1):62-66.

Barr, H., I. Koppel, S. Reeves, M. Hammick, and D. Freeth. 2005. *Effective interprofessional education: Argument, assumption, and evidence.* Oxford and Malden: Blackwell Publishing.

Bates, R. 2004. A critical analysis of evaluation practice: The Kirkpatrick model and the principle of beneficence. *Evaluation and Program Planning* 27:341-347.

Buring, S. M., A. Bhushan, A. Broeseker, S. Conway, W. Duncan-Hewitt, L. Hansen, and S. Westberg. 2009. Interprofessional education: Definitions, student competencies, and guidelines for implementation. *The American Journal of Pharmaceutical Education* 73(4):59.

Cervero, R. M., and J. K. Gaines. 2014. *Effectiveness of continuing medical education: Updated syntheses of systematic reviews*. Chicago, IL: Accreditation Council for Continuing Medical Education.

CIHC (Canadian Interprofessional Health Collaborative). 2010. *A national interprofessional competency framework*. Vancouver, BC: CIHC.

Curtin University. 2011. *Curtin interprofessional capability framework, Sydney, Australia*. http://healthsciences.curtin.edu.au/local/docs/IP_Capability_Framework_booklet.pdf (accessed December 29, 2014).

D'Amour, D., and I. Oandasan. 2004. IECPCP framework. In *Interdisciplinary Education for Collaborative, Patient-Centred Practice: Research and Findings Report*, edited by I. Oandasan, D. D'Amour, M. Zwarenstein, K. Barker, M. Purden, M.-D. Beaulieu, S. Reeves, L. Nasmith, C. Bosco, L. Ginsburg, and D. Tregunno. Ottawa, Canada: Health Canada. http://www.ferasi.umontreal.ca/eng/07_info/IECPCP_Final_Report.pdf (accessed March 17, 2015).

Davis, D., M. O'Brien, N. Freemantle, F. M. Wolf, P. Mazmanian, and A. Taylor-Vaisey. 1999. Impact of formal continuing medical education: Do conferences, workshops, rounds, and other traditional continuing education activities change physician behavior or health care outcomes? *Journal of the American Medical Association* 282(9):867-874.

deBurca, S. 2000. The learning health care organization. *International Journal for Quality in Health Care* 12(6):457-458.

Department of Vermont Health Access. 2014. *Vermont blueprint for health: 2013 annual report (January 30, 2014)*. Williston, VT: Department of Vermont Health Access.

Dow, A., D. Diaz Granados, P. E. Mazmanian, and S. M. Retchin. 2014. An exploratory study of an assessment tool derived from the competencies of the interprofessional education collaborative. *Journal of Interprofessional Care* 28(4):299-304.

Eraut, M. 2004. Informal learning in the workplace. *Studies in Continuing Education* 26(2):247-273.

Fihn, S. D., J. Francis, C. Clancy, C. Nielson, K. Nelson, J. Rumsfeld, T. Cullen, J. Bates, and G. L. Graham. 2014. Insights from advanced analytics at the Veterans Health Administration. *Health Affairs (Millwood)* 33(7):1203-1211.

Forsetlund, L., A. Bjorndal, A. Rashidian, G. Jamtvedt, M. A. O'Brien, F. Wolf, D. Davis, J. Odgaard-Jensen, and A. D. Oxman. 2009. Continuing education meetings and workshops: Effects on professional practice and health care outcomes. *Cochrane Database of Systematic Reviews* 2:Cd003030.

Freeth, D., M. Hammick, S. Reeves, I. Koppel, and H. Barr. 2005a. *Effective interprofessional education: Development, delivery and evaluation*. Oxford: Blackwell Publishing, Ltd.

Freeth, D., S. Reeves, I. Koppel, M. Hammick, and H. Barr. 2005b. *Evaluating interprofessional education: A self-help guide*. London: Higher Education Academy Health Sciences and Practice Network.

Gillan, C., E. Lovrics, E. Halpern, D. Wiljer, and N. Harnett. 2011. The evaluation of learner outcomes in interprofessional continuing education: A literature review and an analysis of survey instruments. *Medical Teacher* 33(9):e461-e470.

Gilman, S. C., D. A. Chokshi, J. L. Bowen, K. W. Rugen, and M. Cox. 2014. Connecting the dots: Interprofessional health education and delivery system redesign at the veterans health administration. *Academic Medicine* 89(8):1113-1116.

Goldman, J., M. Zwarenstein, O. Bhattacharyya, and S. Reeves. 2009. Improving the clarity of the interprofessional field: Implications for research and continuing interprofessional education. *Journal of Continuing Education in the Health Professions* 29(3):151-156.

Gruppen, L. D., R. S. Mangrulkar, and J. C. Kolars. 2012. The promise of competency-based education in the health professions for improving global health. *Human Resources for Health* 10(1):43.

Grymonpre, R., C. van Ineveld, M. Nelson, F. Jensen, A. De Jaeger, T. Sullivan, L. Weinberg, J. Swinamer, and A. Booth. 2010. See it–do it–learn it: Learning interprofessional collaboration in the clinical context. *Journal of Research in Interprofessional Practice and Education* 1(2):127-144.

Hammick, M., D. Freeth, I. Koppel, S. Reeves, and H. Barr. 2007. A best evidence systematic review of interprofessional education: BEME guide no. 9. *Medical Teacher* 29(8):735-751.

Hawkes, G., I. Nunney, and S. Lindqvist. 2013. Caring for attitudes as a means of caring for patients improving medical, pharmacy and nursing student's attitudes to each other's professions by engaging them in interprofessional learning. *Medical Teacher* 35(7):e1302-e1308.

Healthcare Workforce Partnership of Western Mass. n.d. *Healthcare workforce partnership of Western Mass website: Health educators.* http://westernmasshealthcareers.org/local-careers/office-research/health-educators (accessed January 27, 2015).

IOM (Institute of Medicine). 2010. *Redesigning continuing education in the health professions.* Washington, DC: The National Academies Press.

IPEC (Interprofessional Education Collaborative). 2011. *Core competencies for interprofessional collaborative practice: Report of an expert panel.* Washington, DC: IPEC.

Jones, C., and R. Lunge. 2014. *Blueprint for health report: Medical homes, teams, and community health systems.* Montpelier, VT: State of Vermont Agency of Administration Health Care Reform.

Josiah Macy Jr. Foundation. 2010. *Lifelong learning in medicine and nursing: Final conference report.* New York: Josiah Macy Jr. Foundation.

Kirkpatrick, D. L. 1959. Techniques for evaluating training programs. *Journal of American Society of Training Directors* 13(11):3-9.

Kirkpatrick, D. L. 1967. Evaluation of training. In *Training and development handbook,* edited by R. L. Craig and L. R. Bittel. New York: McGraw-Hill. Pp. 87-112.

Kirkpatrick, D. L. 1994. *Evaluating training programs: The four levels.* 1st ed. San Francisco, CA: Berrett-Koehler Publishers, Inc.

Kitto, S., J. Goldman, M. H. Schmitt, and C. A. Olson. 2014. Examining the intersections between continuing education, interprofessional education and workplace learning. *Journal of Interprofessional Care* 28(3):183-185.

Lloyd, B., D. Pfeiffer, J. Dominish, G. Heading, D. Schmidt, and A. McCluskey. 2014. The New South Wales Allied Health Workplace Learning Study: Barriers and enablers to learning in the workplace. *BMC Health Services Research* 14:134.

Marsick, V. J., and M. Volpe. 1999. The nature and need for informal learning. *Advances in Developing Human Resources* 1(3):1-9.

Miller, G. E. 1990. The assessment of clinical skills/competence/performance. *Academic Medicine* 9(Suppl.):S63-S67.

Moore, D. E., Jr., J. S. Green, and H. A. Gallis. 2009. Achieving desired results and improved outcomes: Integrating planning and assessment throughout learning activities. *Journal of Continuing Education in the Health Professions* 29(1):1-15.

Mosley, C., C. Dewhurst, S. Molloy, and B. N. Shaw. 2012. What is the impact of structured resuscitation training on healthcare practitioners, their clients and the wider service? A BEME systematic review: BEME guide no. 20. *Medical Teacher* 34(6):e349-e385.

Mulder, H., O. ten Cate, R. Daalder, and J. Berkvens. 2010. Building a competency-based workplace curriculum around entrustable professional activities: The case of physician assistant training. *Medical Teacher* 32(10):e453-e459.

Nisbet, G., G. D. Hendry, G. Rolls, and M. J. Field. 2008. Interprofessional learning for pre-qualification health care students: An outcomes-based evaluation. *Journal of Interprofessional Care* 22(1):57-68.

Nisbet, G., M. Lincoln, and S. Dunn. 2013. Informal interprofessional learning: An untapped opportunity for learning and change within the workplace. *Journal of Interprofessional Care* 27(6):469-475.

Nowlen, P. M. 1988. *A new approach to continuing education for business and the professions.* New York: Macmillan.

Oandasan, I., and S. Reeves. 2005. Key elements for interprofessional education. Part 2: Factors, processes and outcomes. *Journal of Interprofessional Care* 19(Suppl. 1):39-48.

Owen, J., and M. Schmitt. 2013. Integrating interprofessional education into continuing education: A planning process for continuing interprofessional education programs. *Journal of Continuing Education in the Health Professions* 33(2):109-117.

Purden, M. 2005. Cultural considerations in interprofessional education and practice. *Journal of Interprofessional Care* 19(Suppl. 1):224-234.

Reeves, S., J. Goldman, J. Gilbert, J. Tepper, I. Silver, E. Suter, and M. Zwarenstein. 2011. A scoping review to improve conceptual clarity of interprofessional interventions. *Journal of Interprofessional Care* 25(3):167-174.

Reeves, S., L. Perrier, J. Goldman, D. Freeth, and M. Zwarenstein. 2013. Interprofessional education: Effects on professional practice and healthcare outcomes (update). *Cochrane Database of Systematic Reviews* 3:CD002213.

Reeves, S., S. Boet, B. Zierler, and S. Kitto. 2015. Interprofessional education and practice guide no. 3: Evaluating interprofessional education. *Journal of Interprofessional Care* 29(4):305-312.

Regehr, G., and M. Mylopoulos. 2008. Maintaining competence in the field: Learning about practice, through practice, in practice. *Journal of Continuing Education in the Health Professions* 28(Suppl. 1):S19-S23.

Robben, S., M. Perry, L. van Nieuwenhuijzen, T. van Achterberg, M. O. Rikkert, H. Schers, M. Heinen, and R. Melis. 2012. Impact of interprofessional education on collaboration attitudes, skills, and behavior among primary care professionals. *Journal of Continuing Education in the Health Professions* 32(3):196-204.

Schmitt, M., A. Blue, C. A. Aschenbrener, and T. R. Viggiano. 2011. Core competencies for interprofessional collaborative practice: Reforming health care by transforming health professionals' education. *Academic Medicine* 86(11):1351.

SocialWorkLicensure.org. 2015. *Social work licensure requirements.* http://www.socialwork licensure.org (accessed January 27, 2015).

ten Cate, O. 2013. Nuts and bolts of entrustable professional activities. *Journal of Graduate Medical Education* 5(1):157-158.

Teunissen, P. W., and T. Dornan. 2008. Lifelong learning at work. *BMJ* 336(7645):667-669.

Theilen, U., P. Leonard, P. Jones, R. Ardill, J. Weitz, D. Agrawal, and D. Simpson. 2013. Regular in situ simulation training of paediatric medical emergency team improves hospital response to deteriorating patients. *Resuscitation* 84(2):218-222.

U.S. Department of Labor Bureau of Labor Statistics. 2014. *How to Become a Health Educator or Community Health Worker.* http://www.bls.gov/ooh/community-and-social-service/health-educators.htm#tab-4 (accessed June 5, 2015).

Wagner, S., and S. Reeves. 2015. Milestones and entrustable professional activities: The key to practically translating competencies for interprofessional education? *Journal of Interprofessional Care* 1-2.

Weaver, S. J., and M. A. Rosen. 2013. Team-training in health care: Brief update review. In *Making health care safer II: An updated critical analysis of the evidence for patient safety practices (evidence reports/technology assessments, no. 211).* Rockville, MD: Agency for Healthcare Research and Quality. Pp. 472-479.

WHO (World Health Organization). 2010. *Framework for action on interprofessional education and collaborative practice.* http://www.who.int/hrh/resources/framework_action/en/index.html (accessed March 4, 2013).

Yardley, S., and T. Dornan. 2012. Kirkpatrick's levels and education "evidence." *Medical Education* 46(1):97-106.

4

Strengthening the Evidence Base

Over the past few years, a growing body of work has shown that interprofessional education (IPE) can improve learners' perceptions of interprofessional practice and enhance collaborative knowledge and skills (IOM, 2010; Paradis and Reeves, 2013; Reeves et al., 2011; Remington et al., 2006; Stone, 2006; Thistlethwaite, 2012; Zwarenstein et al., 2009). In contrast, establishing a direct cause-and-effect relationship between IPE and patient, population, and system outcomes has proven more difficult (Brashers et al., 2001; see also Appendixes A and B). It should be emphasized, however, that the evidence directly linking *any* health professions education intervention with individual, population, and system outcomes is far from convincing (Chen et al., 2004; Forsetlund et al., 2009; Lowrie et al., 2014; Marinopoulos et al., 2007; Swing, 2007).

The lack of a well-established causal relationship between IPE and health and system outcomes is due in part to the complexity of the environment in which education interventions are conducted. Generating evidence is difficult even in well-resourced settings; it is even more difficult in parts of the world with fewer research and data resources (Price, 2005; Weaver et al., 2011). The lack of alignment between education and practice (see Chapter 2), the lack of a commonly agreed-upon taxonomy and conceptual model linking education interventions to specific outcomes (see Chapter 3), and the

> "The lack of a well-established causal relationship between IPE and health and system outcomes is due in part to the complexity of the environment in which education interventions are conducted."

relatively long lag time between education interventions and health and system outcomes are major reasons for the paucity of convincing evidence. Other factors include the existence of multiple and often opaque payment structures and a plethora of confounding variables. At the same time, inconsistencies in study designs and methods and a lack of full reporting on the methods employed limit the applicability and generalizability of many research findings (Abu-Rish et al., 2012; Cooper et al., 2001; Olson and Bialocerkowski, 2014; Reeves et al., 2011, 2013; Remington et al., 2006; Salas et al., 2008a; Weaver et al., 2010; Zwarenstein et al., 2009).

With these considerations in mind, the committee commissioned a paper to examine the most current literature linking IPE to health and system outcomes (see Appendix A). Brashers and colleagues explored the challenges of conducting high-quality research in this area, focusing on papers contained in a Cochrane review (Reeves et al., 2013) and studies published between January 2011 and July 2014. After examining more than 2,000 abstracts, they identified 39 studies that met their inclusion criteria, including the 15 studies initially identified in the 2013 Cochrane review. To supplement this work, a group of committee members examined reviews published after a prior article considering the "meta-evidence" for the effects of IPE on patient, population, and system outcomes (Reeves et al., 2010; see Appendix B). They searched PubMed for reviews published from 2010 to 2014 and identified 16 reviews, 8 of which met their inclusion criteria. This chapter draws heavily on the evidence detailed in both of these background papers.

METHODOLOGICAL CHALLENGES

Quantitative, experimental study designs may have limited utility for measuring the effects of IPE on individual, population, and system outcomes. For example, while the committee does not dispute the value of designs such as randomized controlled trials (RCTs) in supporting causal inference, this method has certain limitations for studying the impact of education interventions in general and IPE in particular. Some of these constraints are mentioned by Brashers and colleagues in their background paper (see Appendix A) and are addressed in more detail by Sullivan (2011). In essence, any tightly controlled study design presents challenges for use in studying IPE because the environments in which IPE occurs are highly variable and complex, and the selection of meaningful control groups is problematic (Reeves et al., 2013). Ideally, the control group would receive the same education as the intervention group, but in a uniprofessional manner (Reeves et al., 2009); however, this is rarely feasible.

Table 4-1 contrasts a variety of quantitative study designs with a mixed-methods approach, showing the strengths and limitations of each (Reeves et

TABLE 4-1 Types of Evaluation Design

Qualitative			
Design Type	Description	Strengths	Limitations
Ethnography	This approach entails studying the nature of social interactions, behaviors, and perceptions that occur within teams, organizations, networks, and communities. The central aim of ethnography is to provide rich, holistic insights into people's views and actions, as well as the nature of the location they inhabit, through the collection of detailed observations and interviews.	Generates detailed accounts of actual interactive processes from observational work	Time-consuming and expensive
Grounded theory	This approach is used to explore social processes that present within human interactions. Grounded theory differs from other approaches in that its primary purpose is to develop a theory about dominant social processes rather than to describe particular phenomena. Researchers develop explanations of key social processes that are grounded in or derived from the data.	Provides rich data; can generate new theoretical insight	Development of "micro" theories with limited generalizability
Phenomenology	Phenomenology allows for the exploration and description of phenomena important to the developers of or participants in an activity. The goal is to describe lived experience. Phenomenology is therefore the study of "essences."	Provides rich and detailed descriptions of human lived experience	Focus on a very small number of individuals can generate concerns about limited transferability of findings

continued

TABLE 4-1 Continued

Design Type	Description	Strengths	Limitations
Action research	This approach is known by various names, including "cooperative learning," "participatory action research," and "collaborative research." The research is focused on people involved in a process of change that is the result of a professional, organizational, or community activity. It adopts a more collaborative approach than the designs described above, whereby evaluators play a key role with participants in the processes of planning, implementing, and evaluating the change linked to an activity.	Empowers research participants to make changes in practice	Difficult and time-consuming; typically smaller-scale methods (single case study)
Quantitative			
Design Type	Description	Strengths	Limitations
Randomized controlled trials (RCTs)	In this type of design, participants are randomly selected for inclusion in either intervention or control groups. RCTs can provide a rigorous understanding of causality.	Randomization of individuals reduces bias related to selection or recruitment	Findings are difficult to generalize to those who do not meet the selection criteria (subjects do not represent the larger population)
Controlled before-and-after studies	The approach is similar to an RCT design, but does not entail randomizing who receives the intervention.	Can robustly measure change, but lacks rigor because of the lack of randomization	Cannot be used to evaluate whether reported outcomes are sustained over time

TABLE 4-1 Continued

Design Type	Description	Strengths	Limitations
Interrupted time series studies	This nonrandomized design uses multiple measurements before and after an intervention to determine whether it has an effect that is greater than the underlying trend. This design usually requires multiple time points before the intervention to identify any underlying trends or cyclical phenomena, and multiple points after the intervention to determine whether there has been any change in the trend measured previously.	Allows for statistical investigation of potential biases in estimates of the effect of the intervention; strengthens before-and-after designs (measuring multiple time periods)	Does not control for outside influences on outcomes; also difficult to undertake in settings where routine outcome data are not collected
Before-and-after studies	This is a nonrandomized design in which the evaluator collects data before and after an intervention through the use of surveys.	Helps detect changes resulting from the intervention as data are collected at two points in time: before and after the intervention	Difficult to detect accurately whether any change is attributable to the intervention or another confounding influence

Mixed Methods			
Design Type	Description	Strengths	Limitations
Mixed methods	These designs entail gathering different types of quantitative and qualitative data (e.g., from surveys, interviews, documents, observations) to provide a detailed understanding of processes and outcomes. There are two main types: *sequential* (where data are gathered and analyzed in different stages) and *convergent* (where data are combined together).	Triangulation of quantitative and qualitative data can help generate more insightful findings	Combining different data sets when using a convergent design is methodologically challenging

SOURCE: Adapted from Reeves et al., 2015. For more information, visit http://tandfonline.com/loi/ijic.

al., 2015). However, relatively few studies of IPE have employed qualitative designs or realist approaches to address important contextual issues and confounding factors or variables. While quantitative outcomes are important, such studies can describe only *what* has occurred; they cannot provide an empirical account of *how* or *why* the outcomes were produced. A mixed-methods approach that combines qualitative and quantitative outcomes (see Chapter 5) can offer much more nuanced explanations of IPE interventions.

"Relatively few studies of IPE have employed qualitative designs or realist approaches to address important contextual issues and confounding factors or variables."

Well-designed IPE studies may also be cost-prohibitive (Sullivan, 2011; Swing, 2007). Cost is believed to be the main reason behind the particularly scarce evidence for the effectiveness of IPE in developing countries, although insufficient curriculum integration and a lack of strong leadership may also pose significant challenges (Reed et al., 2005; Sunguya et al., 2014). As a result, the World Health Organization (WHO) has promoted IPE in developing countries based on evidence derived from developed countries; however, the transferability of this evidence may be suspect given the significant differences in their education and health systems. Even in developed countries, moreover, limited resources for studying the impacts of education have affected how IPE studies are conducted.

AREAS OF NEED

The committee identified four major areas of need in which research could begin to establish a more direct rigorous relationship between IPE and individual, population, and system outcomes: (1) constructing well-designed mixed-methods studies that utilize robust qualitative data as well as validated tools for evaluating IPE outcomes, (2) developing a consistent framework for reporting the methodological details of IPE studies, (3) examining the cost and cost-effectiveness of IPE interventions, and (4) linking IPE with changes in collaborative behavior.

Constructing Well-Designed Studies

Study designs in IPE research have improved progressively over the past decade. As with many of the studies in health professions education, however, a considerable number of IPE studies continue to have methodological limitations. All the reviews discussed in Appendix B cite design or methodological weaknesses in the included studies. A number of studies offer only limited or partial descriptions of the interventions. Moreover, many studies provide little discussion of the methodological limitations of this work. Efforts to detect changes in collaborative behavior are particularly poor, often relying on self-reports by learners themselves (Reeves, 2010).

Vocabulary

The inconsistent vocabulary used to describe collaborative work and its associated learning activities and outcomes is a major problem. Use of particular terms is strongly influenced by funding agencies as grant seekers work to match their words and phrasing with that of the funding organizations, and this is one reason for the varied taxonomy currently in use. More than 20 years ago, Leathard (1994) noted the confused terminology in the IPE literature. She pointed out that while the terms "interdisciplinary" and "interprofesssional" are conceptually distinct, it was not uncommon for them to be used interchangeably. Similar findings continue to be reported (e.g., Thannhauser et al., 2010). Such inconsistency in terminology or vocabulary confounds the search for standard research instruments and relevant published articles.

More recently, Paradis and Reeves (2013) analyzed the literature to evaluate trends in the use of interprofessional-related language in article titles. Employing the search terms "interprofessional," "multiprofessional," "multidisciplinar," "interdisciplinar," "transprofessional," and "transdisciplinary," their query yielded 100,488 articles published between 1970 and 2010. The authors found decreasing use of the terms "multidisciplinary/multidisciplinarity" and "interdisciplinary/interdisciplinarity" since the 1980s, while "interprofessional" grew in popularity starting in the 1990s and has remained the dominant term. They also found that "multiprofessional," "transprofessional," and "transdisciplinary" were never widely used.

Reference Models

The lack of a widely accepted model for describing IPE and its associated learning activities and outcomes is another major problem. Studies rarely are based on an explicit conceptual model, and their design and execution suffer as a result. Moreover, the lack of a standard model hinders comparisons among studies and greatly increases the risk entailed in generalizing results across different environments. This issue is discussed in greater detail in Chapter 3.

Measurement Instruments

In their concept analysis, Olenick and colleagues (2010) explore attributes and characteristics of IPE, which they describe as a "complex concept" that would benefit from greater consistency among educators, professionals, and researchers. Given the numerous IPE studies that have been conducted using instruments that lack documented reliability and validity, it is apparent that much confusion remains over appropriate instruments for measuring IPE. Moreover, poorly defined target endpoints have resulted in an incomplete catalogue of potentially available instruments. The background paper in Appendix A identifies three new RCTs in addition to the seven RCTs described in the 2013 Cochrane review (Reeves et al., 2013), each of which suffers from "difficult-to-measure endpoints" (Hoffman et al., 2014; Nurok et al., 2011; Riley et al., 2011).

In addition, the methods used to study the impact of IPE on health and system outcomes vary greatly. The Canadian Interprofessional Health Collaborative (CIHC, 2009) reviewed the literature for available quantitative tools used to measure outcomes of IPE and collaborative practice and identified 128 tools in 136 articles. They found 119 differently named evaluation instruments or methods reported by 20 IPE and collaborative, patient-centered practice projects. However, many of the included tools had not been validated, and their use in other studies would be problematic. The U.S. National Center for Interprofessional Practice and Education is presently engaged in providing better information on IPE evaluation tools.[1]

Sample Size

IPE studies frequently rely on self-reported data, and are small and insufficiently powered to evaluate specified outcomes. For example, Brandt and colleagues (2014) found that approximately 62 percent of the 133 studies they reviewed had sample sizes smaller than 50.

Control Groups

Most IPE studies are not designed to control for differences between comparison and intervention groups. Others suffer from selective reporting of differences in outcomes. Allocation to groups generally is not concealed, and blinding in the assessment of outcomes is often inadequate.

Intermediate Learning Outcomes

Other methodological limitations include a lack of documentation and measurement of intermediate learning outcomes (see Figure 3-2 in Chapter 3). Without documentation of the application and fidelity of the intervention and of important process variables and proximal outcomes,

---

[1] See https://nexusipe.org/measurement-instruments (accessed November 6, 2015).

studies cannot demonstrate clearly that teamwork training actually results in improved teamwork prior to the assessment of health and system outcomes. Similarly, information often is lacking as to whether those trained together actually work collaboratively in the practice setting.

Population-Based Outcomes

Studies examining the impact of IPE all too often ignore important patient and population outcomes. For example, of 39 papers—drawn from the more than 2,000 reviewed abstracts that met the inclusion criteria of Brashers and colleagues (see Appendix A)—none examined population health or community outcomes, and only 4 reported patient or family satisfaction. Rather, the majority focused on organizational or practice processes, with a few addressing a culture of safety. Similar findings have been reported by others (Reeves et al., 2011, 2013; Thistlethwaite, 2012).

Longitudinal Study Design

Studies that span the education continuum and that follow trainees over time, encompassing classrooms, simulation laboratories, and practice settings, are generally lacking (Deutschlander et al., 2013). While there are numerous publications providing examples of brief interprofessional encounters at the learner level, interventions that look at health and system outcomes require longitudinal designs that are more complex and are therefore undertaken less often (Clifton et al., 2006). The imbalance of short- versus long-term studies is exacerbated by a scarcity of coordinating centers at universities for conducting IPE activities, resulting in a large number of "one-off" IPE events that are then evaluated and published. Overcoming the barriers to longitudinal IPE studies would add immeasurably to the evaluation of the effectiveness of IPE.

Developing a Consistent Reporting Framework

The lack of important methodological details in published studies makes analysis suspect, replicability difficult, and generalizability uncertain. The effect of incomplete reporting on the ability to reach general conclusions is evident from the observations on the quality of evidence made by the authors of the reviews summarized in Table B-2 by Reeves and colleagues (see Appendix B). Likewise, Brashers and colleagues (see Appendix A) rate only 4 of the 39 studies they reviewed as "high," indicating that the researchers used a strong study design that produced consistent, generalizable results.

The lack of methodological details reported in IPE publications may be the result of a weak study design or incomplete recording of information on the education intervention itself. For example, authors sometimes give inadequate descriptions of the study participants (e.g., how many, which professions, levels of training) or the type and quantity ("dose") of the intervention as significant variables influencing outcomes (Reeves et al., 2009). It may also be due to the publishing parameters of journal editors that enforce word limitations (Jha, 2014). The literature would be significantly enhanced by the development of a consistent reporting framework for linking IPE to specific learning, health, and system outcomes.

Examining Cost and Cost-Effectiveness

Efforts increasingly focus on documenting the total cost of health care (e.g., the Health Partners model); however, estimates of the total cost of IPE or education in general are lacking. Of the 39 papers in the review by Brashers and colleagues (Appendix A), only 3 identify efficiencies in care (Banki et al., 2013; Capella et al., 2010; Wolf et al., 2010), and only 1 reports changes in practice costs (Banki et al., 2013). While the latter study notes significant cost reductions, they could not be attributed definitively to the IPE intervention itself.

Thirteen of these 39 papers examine outcomes over many months to several years (Armour Forse et al., 2011; Hanbury et al., 2009; Helitzer et al., 2011; Mayer et al., 2011; Morey et al., 2002; Pettker et al., 2009; Phipps et al., 2012; Pingleton et al., 2013; Rask et al., 2007; Sax et al., 2009; Thompson et al., 2000a,b; Wolf et al., 2010). Although these longer-term studies document effects on provider or patient outcomes, the effects tended to decay over time. Moreover, only 2 of the 39 studies (Hanbury et al., 2009; Pettker et al., 2009) were well designed (interrupted time series methodology), making the collective findings difficult to interpret.

Similar observations are made in the analysis of the 8 IPE reviews, encompassing more than 400 individual studies, summarized by Reeves and colleagues (see Appendix B). Across these studies, most authors report only on short-term impacts on learner attitudes and knowledge following various IPE interventions, and do not provide cost analyses. As a result, understanding of the long-term impact of IPE on both education and health system costs continues to be limited. A PubMed search revealed one study that demonstrated the cost-effectiveness of a Danish interprofessional training unit compared with a conventional ward, with no apparent differences in quality or safety between the two (Hansen et al., 2009).

Likewise, while the U.S.-based Vermont Blueprint for Health[2] has

---

[2] Defined as a "program for integrating a system of health care for patients, improving the health of the overall population, and improving control over health care costs by promoting health maintenance, prevention, and care coordination and management" (Vermont Government, 2015).

linked the introduction of its community-based, patient-centered medical home initiative to cost savings, the relationship between these savings and the training of providers to work in teams is unclear.[3] Similar results are emerging from the U.S.-based Veterans Health Administration's patient-aligned care team initiative, which has documented team-based improvements in system outcomes and costs but has not explicitly examined potential relationships between purposeful training for collaborative practice and these outcomes.

Without well-designed studies addressing cost-effectiveness, it will be challenging to formulate a strong business case for IPE. Developing a financial justification for IPE will require knowing the adequate "dose" of IPE (as described in Chapter 3) and having competency or performance measures with which to determine proficiency. These elements and thus the financial justification would no doubt vary given the broad range of "IPE programs" worldwide. Optimally, the business case would include evidence on the sustainability of IPE interventions; their impact on system outcomes, including organizational and practice changes and health care costs; and the resulting patient and population benefits. However, it is worth noting that complex analyses of this type typically are not being conducted for *any* education reform effort and that IPE should not be held to a unique standard.

CONCLUSION

A comprehensive literature search revealed a dearth of robust studies specifically designed to better link IPE with changes in collaborative behavior or answer key questions about the effectiveness of IPE in improving patient, population, and health system outcomes.

Conclusion 3. More purposeful, well-designed, and thoughtfully reported studies are needed to answer key questions about the effectiveness of IPE in improving performance in practice and health and system outcomes.

Linking IPE with Changes in Collaborative Behavior

An essential intermediate step in linking IPE with health and system outcomes is enhanced collaborative behavior and performance in practice (see "Learning Outcomes" in Figure 3-2 in Chapter 3). While considerable attention has been focused on developing measures of interprofessional collaboration (CIHC, 2012; McDonald et al., 2014; National Center for Inter-

---

[3] Personal communication, C. Jones, Blueprint for Health, Deptment of Vermont Health Access, 2014.

professional Practice and Education, 2013; Reeves et al., 2010; Schmitz and Cullen, 2015), no such measures have as yet been broadly accepted or adopted (Clifton, 2006; Hammick et al., 2007; Thannhauser et al., 2010). In fact, the strong contextual dependence of presently available measures (Valentine et al., 2015; WHO, 2013) limits their application beyond a single study or small group of studies. Differences in setting and patient population, education programs and health care delivery institutions, health care workforce composition and patterns of collaboration, and national education and health care policies create significant complexities in study design and interpretation. To address this deficiency the committee makes the following recommendation:

> "The strong contextual dependence of presently available measures of collaborative behavior limits their application beyond a single or small group of studies."

Recommendation 1: Interprofessional stakeholders, funders, and policy makers should commit resources to a coordinated series of well-designed studies of the association between interprofessional education and collaborative behavior, including teamwork and performance in practice. These studies should be focused on developing broad consensus on how to measure interprofessional collaboration effectively across a range of learning environments, patient populations, and practice settings.

These studies could employ different approaches that might include developing instruments and testing their reliability, validity, and usefulness specific to collaborative practice; conducting head-to-head comparisons of existing instruments within particular contexts; and extending the validation process for an existing "best-in-class" instrument to additional professions, learning environments, patient populations, health care settings, and countries. At a minimum, however, these studies should take into account the intended learner outcomes in the three major components of the education continuum—foundational education, graduate education, and continuing professional development (as noted in the "Learning Continuum" of Figure 3-2). Therefore, each such study should clearly define the intermediate (learner) and more distal (health and system) outcome target(s) of the study—for example, how a particular feature of teamwork might be linked to enhanced performance in practice and how such collaboration might promote a particular health or systems outcome (Baker et al., 2006; Franco et al., 2009; Salas et al., 2008b). This perspective, which is often missing or incompletely specified, is essential to the design of robust evaluations of any education intervention in practice (Marinopoulos et al., 2007; Reeves et al., 2013; Swing, 2007).

Addressing the Areas of Need

Addressing these gaps will entail giving IPE greater priority by forming partnerships among the education, practice, and research communities to design studies that are relevant to patient, population, and health system outcomes. Engaging accreditors, policy makers, and funders in the process could provide additional resources for establishing more robust partnerships. Only by bringing all these constituencies together will a series of well-designed studies emerge.

> "Engaging accreditors, policy makers, and funders in the process could provide additional resources for establishing more robust partnerships."

REFERENCES

Abu-Rish, E., S. Kim, L. Choe, L. Varpio, E. Malik, A. A. White, K. Craddick, K. Blondon, L. Robins, P. Nagasawa, A. Thigpen, L. L. Chen, J. Rich, and B. Zierler. 2012. Current trends in interprofessional education of health sciences students: A literature review. *Journal of Interprofessional Care* 26(6):444-451.

Armour Forse, R., J. D. Bramble, and R. McQuillan. 2011. Team training can improve operating room performance. *Surgery* 150(4):771-778.

Baker, D. P., R. Day, and E. Salas. 2006. Teamwork as an essential component of high-reliability organizations. *Health Services Research* 41(4, Pt. 2):1576-1598.

Banki, F., K. Ochoa, M. E. Carrillo, S. S. Leake, A. L. Estrera, K. Khalil, and H. J. Safi. 2013. A surgical team with focus on staff education in a community hospital improves outcomes, costs and patient satisfaction. *American Journal of Surgery* 206(6):1007-1014; discussion 1014-1015.

Brandt, B., M. N. Lutfiyya, J. A. King, and C. Chioreso. 2014. A scoping review of interprofessional collaborative practice and education using the lens of the triple aim. *Journal of Interprofessional Care* 28(5):393-399.

Brashers, V. L., C. E. Curry, D. C. Harper, S. H. McDaniel, G. Pawlson, and J. W. Ball. 2001. Interprofessional health care education: Recommendations of the National Academies of Practice expert panel on health care in the 21st century. *Issues in Interdisciplinary Care* 3(1):21-31.

Capella, J., S. Smith, A. Philp, T. Putnam, C. Gilbert, W. Fry, E. Harvey, A. Wright, K. Henderson, and D. Baker. 2010. Teamwork training improves the clinical care of trauma patients. *Journal of Surgical Education* 67(6):439-443.

Chen, F. M., H. Bauchner, and H. Burstin. 2004. A call for outcomes research in medical education. *Academic Medicine* 79(10):955-960.

CIHC (Canadian Interprofessional Health Collaborative). 2009. *Program evaluation for interprofessional initiatives: Evaluation instruments/methods of the 20 IECPCP projects. A report from the evaluation subcommittee.* Vancouver, BC: CIHC.

CIHC. 2012. *An inventory of quantitative tools measuring interprofessional education and collaborative practice outcomes.* Vancouver, BC: CIHC.

Clifton, M., C. Dale, and C. Bradshaw. 2006. *The impact and effectiveness of inter-professional education in primary care: An RCN literature review.* London, England: Royal College of Nursing. https://www.rcn.org.uk/__data/assets/pdf_file/0004/78718/003091.pdf (accessed March 17, 2015).

Cooper, H., C. Carlisle, T. Gibbs, and C. Watkins. 2001. Developing an evidence base for inter-disciplinary learning: A systematic review. *Journal of Advanced Nursing* 35(2):228-237.

Deutschlander, S., E. Suter, and R. Grymonpre. 2013. Interprofessional practice education: Is the "interprofessional" component relevant to recruiting new graduates to underserved areas? *Rural Remote Health* 13(4):2489.

Forsetlund, L., A. Bjorndal, A. Rashidian, G. Jamtvedt, M. A. O'Brien, F. Wolf, D. Davis, J. Odgaard-Jensen, and A. D. Oxman. 2009. Continuing education meetings and work-shops: Effects on professional practice and health care outcomes. *Cochrane Database of Systematic Reviews* 2:Cd003030.

Franco, L. M., L. Marquez, K. Ethier, Z. Balsara, and W. Isenhower. 2009. *Results of collab-orative improvement: Effects on health outcomes and compliance with evidence-based standards in 27 applications in 12 countries.* Collaborative Evaluation Series. Prepared by University Research Co., LLC (URC). Bethesda, MD: USAID Health Care Improve-ment Project.

Hammick, M., D. Freeth, I. Koppel, S. Reeves, and H. Barr. 2007. A best evidence sys-tematic review of interprofessional education: BEME guide no. 9. *Medical Teacher* 29(8):735-751.

Hanbury, A., L. Wallace, and M. Clark. 2009. Use of a time series design to test effectiveness of a theory-based intervention targeting adherence of health professionals to a clinical guideline. *British Journal of Health Psychology* 14(Pt. 3):505-518.

Hansen, T. B., F. Jacobsen, and K. Larsen. 2009. Cost effective interprofessional train-ing: An evaluation of a training unit in Denmark. *Journal of Interprofessional Care* 23(3):234-241.

Helitzer, D. L., M. Lanoue, B. Wilson, B. U. de Hernandez, T. Warner, and D. Roter. 2011. A randomized controlled trial of communication training with primary care providers to improve patient-centeredness and health risk communication. *Patient Education and Counseling* 82(1):21-29.

Hoffmann, B., V. Muller, J. Rochon, M. Gondan, B. Muller, Z. Albay, K. Weppler, M. Leifermann, C. Miessner, C. Guthlin, D. Parker, G. Hofinger, and F. M. Gerlach. 2014. Effects of a team-based assessment and intervention on patient safety culture in general practice: An open randomised controlled trial. *BMJ Quality and Safety* 23(1):35-46.

IOM (Institute of Medicine). 2010. *The future of nursing: Leading change, advancing health.* Washington, DC: The National Academies Press.

Jha, K. N. 2014. How to write articles that get published. *Journal of Clinical and Diagnostic Research* 8(9):XG01-XG03.

Leathard, A. 1994. Interprofessional developments in Britain. In *Going inter-professional: Working together for health and welfare,* edited by A. Leathard. London: Brunner-Routledge. Pp. 3-37.

Lowrie, R., S. M. Lloyd, A. McConnachie, and J. Morrison. 2014. A cluster randomised con-trolled trial of a pharmacist-led collaborative intervention to improve statin prescribing and attainment of cholesterol targets in primary care. *PLoS ONE* 9(11):e113370.

Marinopoulos, S. S., T. Dorman, N. Ratanawongsa, L. M. Wilson, B. H. Ashar, J. L. Magaziner, R. G. Miller, P. A. Thomas, G. P. Prokopowicz, R. Qayyum, and E. B. Bass. 2007. *Effectiveness of continuing medical education.* Evidence Report/Technology Assessment No. 149. Rockville, MD: Agency for Healthcare Research and Quality.

Mayer, C. M., L. Cluff, W. T. Lin, T. S. Willis, R. E. Stafford, C. Williams, R. Saunders, K. A. Short, N. Lenfestey, H. L. Kane, and J. B. Amoozegar. 2011. Evaluating efforts to optimize TeamSTEPPS implementation in surgical and pediatric intensive care units. *Joint Commission Journal on Quality and Patient Safety* 37(8):365-374.

McDonald, K. M., E. Schultz, L. Albin, N. Pineda, J. Lonhart, V. Sundaram, C. Smith-Spangler, J. Brustrom, E. Malcolm, L. Rohn, and S. Davies. 2014. *Care coordination measures atlas version 4* (Prepared by Stanford University under subcontract to American Institutes for Research on Contract No. HHSA290-2010-00005I). AHRQ Publication No. 14-0037-EF. Rockville, MD: Agency for Healthcare Research and Quality. http://www.ahrq.gov/professionals/prevention-chronic-care/improve/coordination/atlas2014 (accessed April 9, 2015).

Morey, J. C., R. Simon, G. D. Jay, R. L. Wears, M. Salisbury, K. A. Dukes, and S. D. Berns. 2002. Error reduction and performance improvement in the emergency department through formal teamwork training: Evaluation results of the MedTeams project. *Health Services Research Journal* 37(6):1553-1581.

National Center for Interprofessional Practice and Education. 2013. *Measurement instruments*. https://nexusipe.org/measurement-instruments (accessed April 9, 2015).

Nurok, M., L. A. Evans, S. Lipsitz, P. Satwicz, A. Kelly, and A. Frankel. 2011. The relationship of the emotional climate of work and threat to patient outcome in a high-volume thoracic surgery operating room team. *BMJ Quality and Safety* 20(3):237-242.

Olenick, M., L. R. Allen, and R. A. Smego, Jr. 2010. Interprofessional education: A concept analysis. *Advances in Medical Education and Practice* 1:75-84.

Olson, R., and A. Bialocerkowski. 2014. Interprofessional education in allied health: A systematic review. *Medical Education* 48(3):236-246.

Paradis, E., and S. Reeves. 2013. Key trends in interprofessional research: A macrosociological analysis from 1970 to 2010. *Journal of Interprofessional Care* 27(2):113-122.

Pettker, C. M., S. F. Thung, E. R. Norwitz, C. S. Buhimschi, C. A. Raab, J. A. Copel, E. Kuczynski, C. J. Lockwood, and E. F. Funai. 2009. Impact of a comprehensive patient safety strategy on obstetric adverse events. *American Journal of Obstetrics and Gynecology* 200(5):492.e1-492.e8.

Phipps, M. G., D. G. Lindquist, E. McConaughey, J. A. O'Brien, C. A. Raker, and M. J. Paglia. 2012. Outcomes from a labor and delivery team training program with simulation component. *American Journal of Obstetrics and Gynecology* 206(1):3-9.

Pingleton, S. K., E. Carlton, S. Wilkinson, J. Beasley, T. King, C. Wittkopp, M. Moncure, and T. Williamson. 2013. Reduction of venous thromboembolism (VTE) in hospitalized patients: Aligning continuing education with interprofessional team-based quality improvement in an academic medical center. *Academic Medicine* 88(10):1454-1459.

Price, J. 2005. Complexity and interprofessional education. In *The theory-practice relationship in interprofessional education*, Ch. 8, edited by H. Colyer, M. Helme, and I. Jones. King's College, London: Higher Education Academy. Pp. 79-87.

Rask, K., P. A. Parmelee, J. A. Taylor, D. Green, H. Brown, J. Hawley, L. Schild, H. S. Strothers III, and J. G. Ouslander. 2007. Implementation and evaluation of a nursing home fall management program. *Journal of the American Geriatric Society* 55(3):342-349.

Reed, D. A., D. E. Kern, R. B. Levine, and S. M. Wright. 2005. Costs and funding for published medical education research. *Journal of the American Medical Association* 294(9):1052-1057.

Reeves, S. 2010. Ideas for the development of the interprofessional field. *Journal of Interprofessional Care* 24(3):217-219.

Reeves, S., M. Zwarenstein, J. Goldman, H. Barr, D. Freeth, M. Hammick, and I. Koppel. 2009. Interprofessional education: Effects on professional practice and health care outcomes (review). *Cochrane Database Systematic Reviews* (1):1-21.

Reeves, S., J. Goldman, A. Burton, and B. Sawatzky-Girling. 2010. Synthesis of systematic review evidence of interprofessional education. *Journal of Allied Health* 39(Suppl. 1):198-203.

Reeves, S., J. Goldman, J. Gilbert, J. Tepper, I. Silver, E. Suter, and M. Zwarenstein. 2011. A scoping review to improve conceptual clarity of interprofessional interventions. *Journal of Interprofessional Care* 25(3):167-174.

Reeves, S., L. Perrier, J. Goldman, D. Freeth, and M. Zwarenstein. 2013. Interprofessional education: Effects on professional practice and healthcare outcomes (update). *Cochrane Database of Systematic Reviews* 3.

Reeves, S., S. Boet, B. Zierler, and S. Kitto. 2015. Interprofessional education and practice guide no. 3: Evaluating interprofessional education. *Journal of Interprofessional Care* 29 (4):305-312.

Remington, T. L., M. A. Foulk, and B. C. Williams. 2006. Evaluation of evidence for interprofessional education. *The American Journal of Pharmaceutical Education* 70(3):66.

Riley, W., S. Davis, K. Miller, H. Hansen, F. Sainfort, and R. Sweet. 2011. Didactic and simulation nontechnical skills team training to improve perinatal patient outcomes in a community hospital. *Joint Commission Journal on Quality and Patient Safety* 37(8):357-364.

Salas, E., D. DiazGranados, C. Klein, C. S. Burke, K. C. Stagl, G. F. Goodwin, and S. M. Halpin. 2008a. Does team training improve team performance? A meta-analysis. *Human Factors: The Journal of the Human Factors and Ergonomics Society* 50(6):903-933.

Salas, E., N. J. Cooke, and M. A. Rosen. 2008b. On teams, teamwork, and team performance: Discoveries and developments. *Human Factors: The Journal of the Human Factors and Ergonomics Society* 50(3):540-547.

Sax, H. C., P. Browne, R. J. Mayewski, R. J. Panzer, K. C. Hittner, R. L. Burke, and S. Coletta. 2009. Can aviation-based team training elicit sustainable behavioral change? *Archives of Surgery* 144(12):1133-1137.

Schmitz, C. C., and M. J. Cullen. 2015. *Evaluating interprofessional education and collaborative practice: What should I consider when selecting a measurement tool?* https://nexusipe.org/evaluating-ipecp (accessed April 9, 2015).

Stone, N. 2006. Evaluating interprofessional education: The tautological need for interdisciplinary approaches. *Journal of Interprofessional Care* 20(3):260-275.

Sullivan, G. M. 2011. Getting off the "gold standard": Randomized controlled trials and education research. *Journal of Graduate Medical Education* 3(3):285-289.

Sunguya, B. F., M. Jimba, J. Yasuoka, and W. Hinthong. 2014. Interprofessional education for whom?: Challenges and lessons learned from its implementation in developed countries and their application to developing countries: A systematic review. *PLoS ONE* 9(5):e96724.

Swing, S. R. 2007. The ACGME outcome project: Retrospective and prospective. *Medical Teacher* 29(7):648-654.

Thannhauser, J., S. Russell-Mayhew, and C. Scott. 2010. Measures of interprofessional education and collaboration. *Journal of Interprofessional Care* 24(4):336-349.

Thistlethwaite, J. 2012. Interprofessional education: A review of context, learning and the research agenda. *Medical Education* 46(1):58-70.

Thompson, C., A. L. Kinmonth, L. Stevens, R. C. Peveler, A. Stevens, K. J. Ostler, R. M. Pickering, N. G. Baker, A. Henson, J. Preece, D. Cooper, and M. J. Campbell. 2000a. Effects of a clinical-practice guideline and practice-based education on detection and outcome of depression in primary care: Hampshire depression project randomised controlled trial. *Lancet* 355(9199):185-191.

Thompson, R. S., F. P. Rivara, D. C. Thompson, W. E. Barlow, N. K. Sugg, R. D. Maiuro, and D. M. Rubanowice. 2000b. Identification and management of domestic violence: A randomized trial. *American Journal of Preventive Medicine* 19(4):253-263.

Valentine, M. A., I. M. Nembhard, and A. C. Edmondson. 2015. Measuring teamwork in health care settings: A review of survey instruments. *Medical Care* 53(4):e16-e30.

Vermont Government. 2015. *Vermont Government website: New reports show Blueprint is lowering health care costs.* http://governor.vermont.gov/node/2223 (accessed March 17, 2015).

Weaver, L., A. McMurtry, J. Conklin, S. Brajtman, and P. Hall. 2011. Harnessing complexity science for interprofessional education development: A case study. *Journal of Research in Interprofessional Practice and Education* 2(1):100-120.

Weaver, S. J., M. A. Rosen, D. DiazGranados, E. H. Lazzara, R. Lyons, E. Salas, S. A. Knych, M. McKeever, L. Adler, M. Barker, and H. B. King. 2010. Does teamwork improve performance in the operating room? A multilevel evaluation. *Joint Commission Journal on Quality and Patient Safety* 36(3):133-142.

WHO (World Health Organization). 2013. *Interprofessional collaborative practice in primary health care: Nursing and midwifery perspectives. Six case studies.* Geneva: WHO.

Wolf, F. A., L. W. Way, and L. Stewart. 2010. The efficacy of medical team training: Improved team performance and decreased operating room delays: A detailed analysis of 4863 cases. *Annals of Surgery* 252(3):477-483.

Zwarenstein, M., J. Goldman, and S. Reeves. 2009. Interprofessional collaboration: Effects of practice-based interventions on professional practice and healthcare outcomes. *Cochrane Database of Systematic Reviews* 3:CD000072.

5

Improving Research Methodologies

Previous chapters have identified three major barriers to the maturation of interprofessional education (IPE) and collaborative practice: lack of alignment between education and practice (see Chapter 2), lack of a standardized model of IPE across the education continuum (see Chapter 3), and significant gaps in the evidence linking IPE to collaborative practice and patient outcomes (see Chapter 4). This chapter presents the committee's analysis of how best to improve the evidence base and move the field forward.

ENGAGING TEAMS FOR EVALUATION OF IPE

Collaboration is at the heart of effective IPE and interprofessional practice. Likewise, researchers and educators working effectively together in teams could provide a solid foundation on which to build IPE evaluation. As noted in Chapter 4, evaluation of IPE interventions with multiple patient, population, and system outcomes is a complex undertaking. Individuals working alone rarely have the broad evaluation expertise and resources to develop or implement the protocols required to address the key questions in the field (Adams and Dickinson, 2010; ANCC, 2014; Ridde et al., 2009; Turnbull et al., 1998). In the absence of robust research designs, there is a risk that future studies testing the impact of IPE on individual, population, and system outcomes will continue to be unknowingly biased, underpowered to measure true differences, and not generalizable across different systems and types and levels of learners. One possible root cause of poorly designed studies may be that the studies are led by educators who have limited time to devote to research or who may not have formal research training. Therefore, teams of individuals with complementary expertise would be far preferable and have greater impact on measuring the effectiveness of IPE. An IPE evaluation team might include an educational evaluator, a health services researcher, and an economist, in addition to educators and others engaged in IPE.

EMPLOYING A MIXED-METHODS APPROACH

Understanding the full complexity of IPE and the education and health care delivery systems within which it resides is critical for designing studies to measure the impact of IPE on individual, population, and system outcomes. Given this complexity, the use of a single research design or methodology alone may generate findings that fail to provide sufficient detail and context to be informative. IPE research would benefit from the adoption of a mixed-methods approach that combines quantitative and qualitative data to yield insight into both the "what" and "how" of an IPE intervention and its outcomes. Such an approach has been shown to be particularly useful for exploring the perceptions of both individuals and society regarding issues of quality of care and patient safety (Curry et al., 2009; De Lisle, 2011). Creswell and Plano Clark (2007) describe the approach as "a research design with philosophical assumptions as well as methods of inquiry"[1] (p. 5).

The iMpact on practice, oUtcomes and cost of New ROles for health profeSsionals (MUNROS) project (see Box 5-1) is an example of a longitudinal, mixed-methods approach for evaluating the impact of health professional teams organized to deliver services in a more cost-effective manner following the recent financial crisis experienced by most European countries.

Comparative Effectiveness Research

Comparative effectiveness research[2] is one approach for combining different study methods used in complex environments such as health

---

[1] "As a methodology, it involves philosophical assumptions that guide the direction of the collection and analysis of data and the mixture of qualitative and quantitative approaches in many phases in the research process. As a method, it focuses on collecting, analyzing, and mixing both quantitative and qualitative data in a single study or series of studies. Its central premise is that the use of quantitative and qualitative approaches in combination provides a better understanding of research problems than either approach alone" (Creswell and Plano Clark, 2007, p. 5).

[2] The Institute of Medicine (IOM) Committee on Comparative Effectiveness Research Prioritization defines comparative effectiveness research as "the generation and synthesis of evidence that compares the benefits and harms of alternative methods to prevent, diagnose, treat, and monitor a clinical condition or to improve the delivery of care" (IOM, 2010, p. 41).

BOX 5-1
The iMpact on practice, oUtcomes and cost of New ROles for health profeSsionals (MUNROS) Project

With support from the European Commission, the MUNROS project is a 4-year systematic evaluation of the impact of changing health professional roles and team-based delivery of health services (MUNROS, 2015). Universities from nine different European countries make up the consortium designing the cross-sectional and multilevel study. They employ a mixed-methods approach to evaluate the impact of the newly defined professional roles on clinical practice, patient outcomes, health systems, and costs in a range of different health care settings within the European Union and Associate Countries (Czech Republic, England, Germany, Italy, Netherlands, Norway, Poland, Scotland, and Turkey).

The study is divided into 10 research processes as follows:

1 and 2: Develop an evaluation framework for mapping the skills and competencies of the health workforce, which will be used in the economic evaluation of the data.

3: Collect information that can aid in the development of questionnaires for health care professionals, managers, and patients. This is done using case study methodology to identify the contributions of the new health professionals.

4: Develop the questionnaires.

5 and 6: Implement the surveys. The survey of the health professionals is aimed at determining the impact of new professional roles on clinical practice and the organization of care; the survey of patients assesses the impact of the new professionals on patient satisfaction and personal experiences.

7: Collect secondary data on hospital processes, productivity, and health outcomes. The data will be helpful in assessing the impact of the new professionals.

8: Conduct an economic evaluation that includes costs and benefits of the new professional roles and identifies incentives for increasing their impact.

9: Based on the collected data, provide examples of optimal models of integration of care and the associated costs, and offer detail on how the new professional roles might be carried out to improve the integration of care.

10: Build a workforce planning model for all levels of care that reflects the dynamic interaction between the workforce skill mix and the quality and cost of care for patients.

Following analysis of the data on the costs of these newly organized health care teams, European and country-level stakeholders will be engaged to maximize the impact of the results at the policy and practitioner levels.

care that, according to a previous Institute of Medicine (IOM) committee, can "assist consumers, clinicians, purchasers, and policy makers to make informed decisions that will improve health care at both the individual and population levels" (IOM, 2010, p. 41; Sox and Goodman, 2012). An important element of comparative effectiveness research is determining the benefit an intervention produces in routine clinical practice, rather than in a carefully controlled setting. Through such studies, it may also be possible to evaluate the financial justification for IPE—an important part of any return-on-investment analysis, as discussed below.

Return on Investment

Demonstrating financial return on investment is part of comparative effectiveness research and a key element for the sustainability of all health professions education, including IPE (Bicknell et al., 2001; IOM, 2014; Starck, 2005; Walsh et al., 2014). Proof-of-concept studies demonstrating the impact of IPE on individual, population, and systems outcomes, including a return on investment, will likely be necessary if there are to be greater financial investments in IPE. This is where alignment between the education and health care delivery systems becomes critical so that the academic partner (creating the IPE intervention/activity) and care delivery system partner (hosting the intervention and showcasing the outcomes) are working together. High-level stakeholders, such as policy makers, regulatory agencies, accrediting bodies, and professional organizations that oversee or encourage collaborative practice, will need to contribute as well. These stakeholders might, for example, provide incentives for programs and organizations to better align IPE with collaborative practice so the potential long-term savings in health care costs can be evaluated.

> "Demonstrating financial return on investment is part of comparative effectiveness research and a key element for the sustainability of all health professions education, including IPE."

The framework developed by the Canadian Institute on Governance (see Figure 5-1) and described by Nason (2011) and Suter (2014) was created to facilitate analysis of the return on investment of specific IPE interventions or collaborative care approaches. This framework includes a logic model for tracing input costs through to benefits, and although as yet untested, may prove useful as a framework for investigating the return on investment of IPE.

Based on the evidence and the committee's expert opinion, it is apparent that using either quantitative or qualitative methods alone will limit the ability of investigators in both developed and developing countries to

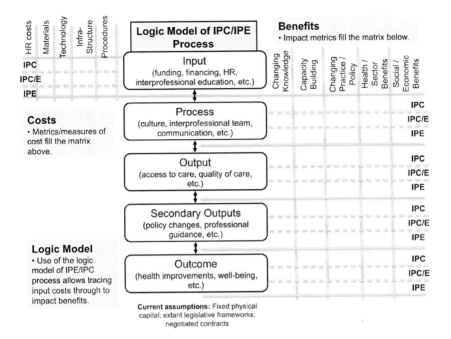

FIGURE 5-1 A framework for analysis of return on investment of IPE interventions or collaborative care approaches.

NOTE: HR = human resources; IPC = interprofessional collaboration; IPE = interprofessional education.

SOURCE: Nason, 2011. Used with kind permission of the Institute on Governance and the Health Education Task Force.

produce high-quality studies linking IPE with health and system outcomes. The committee therefore makes the following recommendation:

> **Recommendation 2: Health professions educators and academic and health system leaders should adopt mixed-methods study designs for evaluating the impact of interprofessional education (IPE) on health and system outcomes. When possible, such studies should include an economic analysis and be carried out by teams of experts that include educational evaluators, health services researchers, and economists, along with educators and others engaged in IPE.**

Once best practices in the design of IPE studies have been established, disseminating them widely through detailed reporting or publishing can strengthen the evidence base and help guide future studies in building on a foundation of high-quality empirical work linking IPE to outcomes. These studies could include those focused on eliciting in-depth patient, family, and caregiver experiences of collaborative practice. Sharing best practices in IPE study design is an important way of improving the quality of studies themselves. Work currently under way on developing methods for evaluating the impact of IPE—such as that of the U.S. National Center for Interprofessional Practice and Education—could inform the work of those with fewer resources provided that the concepts and methodologies employed are used appropriately and adapted to the local context in which they are applied. Box 5-2 offers suggestions for a potential program for evaluative research connecting IPE to health and system outcomes.

CLOSING REMARKS

More robust evaluation designs and methods could increase the number of high-quality IPE studies. The use of a mixed-methods approach would be

---

BOX 5-2
Connecting IPE to Health and System Outcomes:
A Potential Program of Research

A. Identify and Secure Key Program Elements

1. Ensure that education and health system leaders are supportive of the program and that sufficient resources will be available to accomplish and sustain the work (see Chapter 2). Without these elements in place or clearly identified, the feasibility, scope, and substance of the program will be open to question.
2. Assemble an interprofessional evaluation team as early as possible. The design of the evaluation plan should proceed concurrently with the development of the education interventions.
3. Select and be guided by a conceptual model that provides a comprehensive framework encompassing the education continuum; learning, health, and system outcomes; and confounding factors (see Chapter 3).
4. Although classroom and simulation activities are valuable early in the learning continuum, and their evaluation can be informative, the clinical or community workplace is the preferred site for evaluating the effects of IPE on health and system outcomes.
5. Identify workplace learning sites (practice environments) in which interprofessional activities are built on sound theoretical underpinnings and add value to the overall work of the site. Connecting students with team-based quality improvement and patient safety activities may be especially valuable.
6. Learning teams should include the appropriate professions and levels of learners for the clinical tasks required of them and should be adequately prepared for the workplace learning opportunities provided.

particularly useful. Both "big data" and smaller data sources could prove useful if studies are well designed and the outcomes well delineated. It will be important to identify and evaluate collective (i.e., team, group, network) as well as individual outcomes.

In addition and where applicable, the use of randomized and longitudinal designs that are adequately powered could demonstrate differences between groups or changes over time. Using the realist evaluation approach could provide in-depth understanding of IPE interventions beyond outcomes by illuminating how the outcomes were produced, by whom, under what conditions, and in what settings (Pawson and Tilley, 1997). This information could be particularly useful for maximizing resource allocation, which might also be informed through comparative effectiveness research.

Organizing studies to elicit in-depth patient, family, and caregiver experiences related to their involvement in IPE could promote alignment between education and practice to impact person-centered outcomes. A similar design could be used in studying the impact of IPE on specific com-

---

7. Faculty, preceptor, and staff development generally is necessary to ensure positive experiences and exposure of learners to applied interprofessional activities.
8. Ensure that the IPE interventions being evaluated are competency-based and linked to team behaviors that support interprofessional collaborative practice. If this is not the case, preliminary studies should be conducted to establish these relationships.

B. Select a Robust Evaluation Design

1. Select the most robust evaluation methods for the health and system outcomes being addressed. The particular evaluation methods will depend on the specific question(s) being examined, but give serious consideration to using both qualitative and quantitative methods (as described in Table 4-1). Using a single data set can limit the level of detail a study is able to produce. A mixed-methods approach can generate more comprehensive information about an IPE intervention/activity.
2. Randomized controlled trials (RCTs) are still considered the "gold standard" but may not always be feasible in practice settings because of the relatively small numbers of subjects, as well as difficulties in assigning learners to control and intervention groups. Controlled before-and-after studies have similar limitations.
3. In some cases, cluster randomized designs (involving groups of teams or individual practices) can be used to overcome difficulties in assigning subjects to control and intervention groups, but intermixing may still be a problem.
4. Although commonly employed in education research, uncontrolled before-and-after studies generally do not have the power or precision to link education interventions to health and systems outcomes.

munity and public health outcomes to build the evidence base in this area. Studying systems in which best practices in IPE cross the continuum from education to health or health care (e.g., the Veterans Health Administration and countries where education and health ministries work together) could illuminate a path for greater alignment between systems in different settings.

Disseminating best practices through detailed reporting or publishing could also strengthen the evidence base and help guide future research. Both formal publication and informal channels such as blogs and newsletters can be powerful platforms for getting messages to researchers. The use of tools such as Replicability of Interprofessional Education (RIPE) could facilitate greater replicability of IPE studies through more structured and standardized reporting (Abu-Rish et al., 2012). Journal editors might require researchers to publish supplemental details on their IPE interventions and outcomes online, and well-designed and well-executed studies could be used as exemplars on websites. Given time and resource constraints, having access to robust study designs and better descriptions for replicability could greatly assist faculty in meeting IPE accreditation standards. For standardization, research teams could be encouraged to draw on the modified Kirkpatrick typology (Barr et al., 2005) and available toolkits when designing evaluations of IPE interventions. Another resource is the work of Reeves and colleagues (2015), who provide guidance on how to design and implement more robust studies of IPE.

In recognition of the importance of placing individual and population health at the center of health professions education, the committee has offered three major conclusions: (1) on the need for better alignment of education and health care delivery systems, (2) the need for a standardized model of IPE, and (3) the need for a stronger evidence base linking IPE to health and system outcomes. The committee also has put forth two recommendations for consideration by research teams: (1) the development of measures of collaborative performance that are effective across a broad range of learning environments; and (2) the adoption of a mixed-methods approach when evaluating IPE outcomes.

> The committee recognizes "the importance of placing individual and population health at the center of health professions education."

Collectively, these conclusions and recommendations are aimed at elevating the profile of IPE in a rapidly changing world. The committee hopes this report will shed additional light on the value of collaboration among educators, researchers, practitioners, patients, families, and communities, as well as all those who come together in working to improve lives through treatment and palliation, disease prevention, and wellness interventions. Only through the publication of rigorously designed studies can the potential impact of IPE on health and health care be fully realized.

REFERENCES

Abu-Rish, E., S. Kim, L. Choe, L. Varpio, E. Malik, A. A. White, K. Craddick, K. Blondon, L. Robins, P. Nagasawa, A. Thigpen, L. L. Chen, J. Rich, and B. Zierler. 2012. Current trends in interprofessional education of health sciences students: A literature review. *Journal of Interprofessional Care* 26(6):444-451.
Adams, J., and P. Dickinson. 2010. Evaluation training to build capability in the community and public health workforce. *American Journal of Evaluation* 31(3):421-433.
ANCC (American Nurses Credentialing Center). 2014. *The importance of evaluating the impact of continuing nursing education on outcomes: Professional nursing practice and patient care.* Silver Spring, MD: ANCC's Commission on Accreditation.
Barr, H., I. Koppel, S. Reeves, M. Hammick, and D. Freeth. 2005. *Effective interprofessional education: Argument, assumption, and evidence.* Oxford and Malden: Blackwell Publishing.
Bicknell, W. J., A. C. Beggs, and P. V. Tham. 2001. Determining the full costs of medical education in Thai Binh, Vietnam: A generalizable model. *Health Policy and Planning* 16(4):412-420.
Creswell, J. W., and V. L. Plano Clark. 2007. *Designing and conducting mixed methods research.* Thousand Oaks, CA: Sage Publications.
Curry, L. A., I. M. Nembhard, and E. H. Bradley. 2009. Qualitative and mixed methods provide unique contributions to outcomes research. *Circulation* 119(10):1442-1452.
De Lisle, J. 2011. The benefits and challenges of mixing methods and methodologies: Lessons learnt from implementing qualitatively led mixed methods research designs in Trinidad and Tobago. *Caribbean Curriculum* 18:87-120.
IOM (Institute of Medicine). 2010. *Redesigning continuing education in the health professions.* Washington, DC: The National Academies Press.
IOM. 2014. *Graduate medical education that meets the nation's health needs.* Washington, DC: The National Academies Press.
MUNROS (iMpact on practice, oUtcomes and cost of New ROles for health profeSsionals. 2015. *Health care reform: The impact on practice, outcomes and costs of new roles for health professionals.* https://www.abdn.ac.uk/munros (accessed March 17, 2015).
Nason, E. 2011. *The "ROI" in "team": Return on investment analysis framework, indicators and data for IPC and IPE.* Ontario, Canada: Institute on Governance.
Pawson, R., and N. Tilley. 1997. *Realistic evaluation.* London: Sage Publications.
Reeves, S., S. Boet, B. Zierler, and S. Kitto. 2015. Interprofessional education and practice guide no. 3: Evaluating interprofessional education. *Journal of Interprofessional Care* 29(4):305-312.
Ridde, V., P. Fournier, B. Banza, C. Tourigny, and D. Ouedraogo. 2009. Programme evaluation training for health professionals in Francophone Africa: Process, competence acquisition and use. *Human Resources for Health* 7:3.
Sox, H. C., and S. N. Goodman. 2012. The methods of comparative effectiveness research. *Annual Review of Public Health* 33:425-445.
Starck, P. L. 2005. The cost of doing business in nursing education. *Journal of Professional Nursing* 21(3):183-190.

Suter, E. 2014. *Presentation at open session for measuring the impact of interprofessional education (IPE) on collaborative practice and patient outcomes: A consensus study.* http://www.iom.edu/Activities/Global/MeasuringtheImpactofInterprofessionalEducation/2014-OCT-07.aspx (accessed December 8, 2014).

Turnbull, J., J. Gray, and J. MacFadyen. 1998. Improving in-training evaluation programs. *Journal of General Internal Medicine* 13(5):317-323.

Walsh, K., S. Reeves, and S. Maloney. 2014. Exploring issues of cost and value in professional and interprofessional education. *Journal of Interprofessional Care* 28(6):493-494.

Appendix A

Review: Measuring the Impact of Interprofessional Education (IPE) on Collaborative Practice and Patient Outcomes

*Valentina Brashers, M.D.; Elayne Phillips, M.P.H., Ph.D., R.N.;
Jessica Malpass, Ph.D., R.N.; John Owen, Ed.D., M.Sc.*

BACKGROUND

Although the complexity of patient care demands that health care teams collaborate effectively, there remains a paucity of high-quality research that measures the impact of interprofessional education (IPE) on practice processes and patient outcomes. A recent Cochrane review found a total of 15 articles published between 1999 and 2011 whose methodology met their stringent criteria for inclusion (Reeves et al., 2013). While those studies did provide evidence that IPE interventions can produce positive outcomes, there remains a need to identify best practices for research that effectively link IPE interventions with measurable changes in practice processes and patient outcomes.

OBJECTIVES

The two objectives of this review are to

- examine the currently best-available methods used for measuring the impact of IPE on collaborative practice, patient outcomes, or both; and
- describe the challenges to conducting high-quality research that seeks to link IPE interventions with measurable changes in practice and patient outcomes.

METHODS

This review focuses on studies reviewed in the Reeves and colleagues (2013) Cochrane review, and on any national and international studies published from January 2011 to July 2014.

Criteria for Considering Studies for This Review

Types of Studies

This review includes randomized controlled trials (RCTs), controlled before-and-after (CBA) studies, interrupted time series (ITS) studies, and uncontrolled before-and-after (BA) studies.

Types of Participants

This review includes various types of health care professionals (physicians, dentists, chiropractors, midwives, nurses, nurse practitioners, physical therapists, occupational therapists, respiratory therapists, speech and language therapists, pharmacists, technicians, psychotherapists, and social workers).

Types of Interventions

As defined by Reeves and colleagues (2013, p. 5), "An IPE intervention occurs when members of more than one health or social care (or both) profession learn interactively together, for the explicit purpose of improving interprofessional collaboration or the health/well-being (or both) of patients/clients. Interactive learning requires active learner participation, and active exchange between learners from different professions."

Types of Outcome Measures

Outcome measures include

- objectively measured patient/client outcomes (disease incidence; morbidity, mortality, readmission, and complication rates; length of stay; patient/family satisfaction);
- objectively measured health care process measurements (changes in efficiency [resources, time, cost]; teamwork; approach to patient care or follow-up); and
- subjective self-reported outcomes, included only when objective measures were also reported.

Search Methods

For this review, the following search methods were used:

- A search was conducted of Ovid, PubMed, and CINAHL (Cumulative Index to Nursing and Allied Health Literature) via MeSH (Medical Subject Headings) terms "Interprofessional education AND (Cochrane terms OR Quality OR Clinical Outcomes OR Patient Outcomes OR Cost Benefit OR Quality OR Patient Safety OR Patient Satisfaction OR Provider Satisfaction OR Morbidity)" from January 2011 to the present.
- A keyword search from PubMed using "interprofessional education" or "team training" in the title/abstract (limit 2008-July 2014) was also conducted.
- Articles were hand-pulled from the Reeves et al. (2013) Cochrane review.

Data Collection and Analysis

Two of the review authors (EKP and JKM) jointly reviewed 2,347 abstracts retrieved by the searches to identify all those that indicated

- an IPE intervention was implemented;
- health care clinicians of various backgrounds were trained; and
- patient outcomes (patient safety, patient satisfaction, quality of care, cost, clinical outcomes, community health outcomes, etc.) and/or provider outcomes (provider satisfaction, measures of collaborative practice, communication) were reported.

Abstracts were excluded if

- the interprofessional intervention lacked a concrete educational component;
- interprofessional activities involved only students;
- learning outcomes were the only outcomes measured; or
- reported outcomes included only feelings, beliefs, attitudes, or perceptions.

Forty-seven studies were identified from the abstract search as potentially meeting these inclusion criteria. The full text of each of these articles as well as each of the 15 articles pulled from the Cochrane review was independently reviewed by three of the review authors (EKP, JKM, VLB). An appraisal form was developed specifically for this review that evaluated the studies for

- type of study (RCT, CBA, ITS, or BA study with historical control, contemporaneous control, or no control);
- outcome measures;
- outcome tool;
- sample size and composition;
- setting;
- type of IPE intervention; and
- findings (a brief overview of findings is included in a detailed table in the annex at the end of this appendix, but findings are not discussed as part of this review, which is focused on methodology).

These data were entered into a spreadsheet, and any disagreements and uncertainties were resolved by discussion. These studies were then given an overall rating based on the following definitions:

X   Study did not meet inclusion criteria

LEVEL I   RCT or experimental study

LEVEL II   Quasi-experimental (no manipulation of independent variable; may have random assignment or control)

LEVEL III   Nonexperimental (no manipulation of independent variable; includes descriptive, comparative, and correlational studies; uses secondary data)

LEVEL III   Qualitative (exploratory [e.g., interviews, focus groups]; starting point for studies where little research exists; small samples sizes; results used to design empirical studies)

The following descriptions were used as general guidelines for rating:

A - HIGH
- Consistent, generalizable results
- Sufficient sample size
- Adequate control
- Definitive conclusions
- Consistent recommendations based on a comprehensive literature review that includes thorough reference to scientific evidence

B - GOOD
- Reasonably consistent results
- Sufficient sample size for the study design
- Some control
- Fairly definitive conclusions

- Reasonably consistent recommendations based on a fairly comprehensive literature review that includes some reference to scientific evidence

C - LOW
- Little evidence with inconsistent results
- Insufficient sample size for study design
- Conclusions cannot be drawn

MAIN RESULTS

In addition to the 15 studies from the Cochrane review, 24 additional studies met all criteria and were included in this review. Table A-1 presents an overview of the results of the review.

Study Types

Randomized Controlled Trials: Three new RCTs (Hoffmann et al., 2014; Nurok et al., 2011; Riley et al., 2011) were added to the seven RCTs described in the 2013 Cochrane review (Reeves et al., 2013). These three studies suffered from many of the same methodologic limitations noted for the studies discussed in the Cochrane review, such as the lack of concealed allocation, inadequate blinding in the assessment of outcomes, and evidence of selective outcome reporting. These studies were also characterized by additional sources of error that are common in evaluating educational programs (Sullivan, 2011), including differences in the quality of the education intervention (e.g., type of learners trained, variation in learner and instructor experience and training) and difficult-to-measure endpoints.

Controlled Before-and-After Studies: No new CBAs were added during this review. As described in the 2013 Cochrane review, the CBAs were characterized by many of the same limitations described for RCTs, except that there was often a more well-documented effort to ensure that baseline characteristics of the intervention and control groups were similar.

Interrupted Time Series Studies: One additional ITS (Pettker et al., 2009) was added to those listed in the 2013 Cochrane Review. The primary strength of this study was the documentation of long-term changes in outcomes. There was also a sequential introduction of interventions in an effort to isolate the effect of the IPE intervention from numerous other practice changes introduced during the study period. However, while the trend in outcomes was calculated on a monthly basis, it is not clear from the analysis whether the team training alone significantly affected outcome trends.

Before-and-After Studies: The 20 BA studies that were included in this review were carefully chosen for having used credible research methods

TABLE A-1 Overview of Results

Criteria	Results
Type of Study and Rating (n)	• RCT = 10 (IA = 3; IB = 7) • CBA = 6 (IIA = 1; IIB = 5) • ITS = 3 (IIB = 3) • BA = 20 (IIB = 17; IIC = 3)
Outcome Measures: Patients	• Number of adverse events (e.g., thrombosis, premature births, infections) • Quality improvement goals (e.g., hemoglobin A1c test, cholesterol, blood pressure) • Number of falls • Functional improvements • Length of stay • Community discharge (versus to a care facility) • Readmission rates • Clinical improvement (depression) • Morbidity • Mortality • Patient and family satisfaction
Outcome Measures: Practice	• Observed team behaviors • Observed practice competencies (e.g., code team performance, use of checklists, clinical identification of battered women or depression, adherence to national guidelines, quality of management plans) • Organization of care (e.g., community linkages, self-management support, decision support, clinical information system) • Clinical documentation • Provider–patient communication • Observed errors, number of safety events, and frequency of reporting • Time savings (e.g., time to antibiotic administration or surgery case starts, operating room [OR] time, time to initiate urgent care) • Delays in care (e.g., equipment malfunction, OR delays) • Cost savings (e.g., OR costs, hospital room costs)
Patient and Practice Outcome Tools	• Clinical database/chart review • Incidence reports • Clinical performance measures • Standardized practice evaluation tools (e.g., Assessment of Chronic Illness Care, Team Dimension Rating, Competency Assessment Instrument, Surgical Quality Improvement Program Tool, Teamwork Evaluation of Non-Technical Skills, Trauma Team Performance Observation Tool) • Observation of provider performance using self-designed tools • Standardized patient outcome tools (e.g., Weighted Adverse Outcomes Scores, Press Ganey Patient Satisfaction Tool, Family Satisfaction in the intensive care unit (ICU) Tool) • Provider interviews

TABLE A-1 Continued

Criteria	Results
Sample Size and Composition of Providers Trained (when reported)	• Sample Size —Number of providers trained (range 18 to >1,000) —Number of patients assessed (range 21 to >500) —Number of procedures (range 73 to >100,000) • Composition of Providers Trained —All studies included nurses or nurse practitioners —All but two studies included physicians —Four studies reported pharmacist participation —Eight studies reported therapist participation —Nine studies reported technician participation —Four studies reported social worker participation —Other: nutritionist, housekeeping, scheduler, physician assistant, unit secretary, chaplain, psychologist, security officer • Unclear: "ancillary personnel," "support personnel," "OR team," "health care team," and "health care assistants"
Setting (n)	• U.S. Academic Health Centers —Primary care = 2 —General acute care = 1 —ICU = 2; OR = 6 —Emergency department = 3 —Labor and delivery = 2 • U.S. community practices (including mental health clinics) —Primary care = 3 —General acute care = 3 —ICU = 1; OR = 2 —Emergency department = 2 —Labor and delivery = 2 • U.S. Veterans Health Administration = 3 • Other: —U.S. nursing home —U.S. free-standing magnetic resonance imaging (MRI) facility —U.S. combat theater of operations —Mexico: public health center —Britain: primary care clinic = 2 —Britain: academic health center ICU —Britain: National Health Service (NHS) hospital —Germany: general practices
Type of IPE Intervention (n)	• Design —Crew resource management = 9 —TeamSTEPPS (Team Strategies and Tools to Enhance Performance and Patient Safety) = 6 —MedTeams labor and delivery team coordination course = 1 —Emergency team coordination course = 1 —Composite resuscitation team training = 1 —Schwartz rounds = 1 —In-house design = 21 • Format: All included some didactic and discussion; some included Web-based learning; in addition to TeamSTEPPS, four studies included simulations, and three trainings were in situ

continued

TABLE A-1 Continued

Criteria	Results
Findings (n)	• Care Quality —Most studies reported improvements in practice processes —Specific patient care quality outcomes improved = 4 —Overall improved morbidity and mortality = 6 • Patient Safety —Reduction in adverse outcomes mixed = 7 —Error rates reduced = 2 • Patient satisfaction improved = 2 • Care efficiencies or costs improved = 4

NOTE: Detailed results are presented in Annex A-1 at the end of this appendix.

based on our rating scale (i.e., IIB or IIC, as defined earlier). These studies were highly diverse in their outcome measures, measurement tools, setting, number and composition of participants, presence of historical controls, and type and quality of IPE interventions. Two BA studies that were rated IIC were included because of the quality of their design, but their interpretation of the results went beyond what the data could support (Capella et al., 2010; Pingleton et al., 2013). One study rated IIC was included because it was conducted in an unusual but important care setting (Lang et al., 2010).

Outcome Measures

Studies chosen for inclusion in this review reported objective and measurable outcomes. Patient outcome measures addressed many important issues in care quality, such as number of adverse events, specific indices of disease progression, length of stay, improvement in symptoms, morbidity, and mortality as derived from review of the clinical database for BA IPE interventions. Two studies assessed provider-with-patient communication skills (Brown et al., 1999; Helitzer et al., 2011). Only four studies measured patient satisfaction (Banki et al., 2013; Brown et al., 1999; Campbell et al., 2001; Morey et al., 2002), and one measured family satisfaction (Shaw et al., 2014).

Practice outcome measures most often addressed clinical decision making, behaviors related to patient safety, care efficiency, error reporting, adherence to guidelines, use of checklists, organization of care, and specific care competencies. Nine studies included objective observation of teamwork skills in the actual delivery of care (Bliss et al., 2012; Capella et al., 2010; Halverson et al., 2009; Mayer et al., 2011; Morey et al., 2002; Nurok et al., 2011; Patterson et al., 2013; Steinemann et al., 2011; Weaver et al., 2010), and two studies reported observed team behaviors in the simulated setting in addition to the care delivery site (Knight et al., 2014;

Patterson et al., 2013). Only one study directly measured changes in practice costs (Banki et al., 2013).

Several studies measured outcomes over many months and even years to assess for sustained changes in patient or provider outcomes (Armour Forse et al., 2011; Helitzer et al., 2011; Mayer et al., 2011; Morey et al., 2002; Pettker et al., 2009; Phipps et al., 2012; Pingleton et al., 2013; Rask et al., 2007; Sax et al., 2009; Thompson et al., 2000b; Wolf et al., 2010). For these studies, improvements were sustained over the study period, although some reported partial decay over time. Another complication is that while these studies included graphics that listed outcomes at multiple time points before and after the IPE intervention, only two were actual ITS studies (Hanbury et al., 2009; Pettker et al., 2009). One based its conclusions on the single lowest and highest pre- and postintervention values (Pingleton et al., 2013), and the rest based their conclusions on the average of before and after outcomes.

Patient and Practice Outcome Tools

The most commonly used measurement tool for both provider and patient outcomes involved chart review/clinical database access for retrieving specific patient data, error/adverse event/incident reporting, and OR reports. Most observational studies used validated tools such as the Trauma Oxford Non-Technical Skills scale (Steinemann et al., 2011), Teamwork Evaluation of Non-Technical Skills tool (Mayer et al., 2011), American College of Surgeons National Surgical Quality Improvement Program tool (Bliss et al., 2012), Behavioral Markers for Neonatal Resuscitation Scale (Patterson et al., 2013), Medical Performance Assessment Tool for Communication and Teamwork (Weaver et al., 2010), and Trauma Team Performance Observation Tool (Capella et al., 2010). One study used the validated Roter Interaction Analysis System provider–patient communication tool (Helitzer et al., 2011). Shaw and colleagues (2014) used a validated Family Satisfaction in the ICU tool to link teamwork with family-perceived provider communication. Patient satisfaction was measured using the Press Ganey Patient Satisfaction Tool in one study (Banki et al., 2013), and the Patient Safety Satisfaction Survey in another (Campbell et al., 2001). A blended tool taken from several sources was used in one study (Morey et al., 2002), and a tool designed by the researchers was used in another (Brown et al., 1999).

Sample Size and Composition of Providers Trained

All but 3 of the 10 RCTs (Brown et al., 1999; Helitzer et al., 2011; Nurok et al., 2011) and 1 CBA (Weaver et al., 2010) described in this updated review had large sample sizes involving multiple practice sites. For example, one cluster RCT trained more than 1,300 providers whose outcomes were measured in 15 military and civilian hospitals across multiple states (Nielsen et al., 2007). Sample size in the ITS and BA studies varied widely, and several studies failed to report a specific number of participants trained (Armour Forse et al., 2011; Knight et al., 2014; Nurok et al., 2011; Theilen et al., 2013). The composition of providers trained varied significantly. All studies included nurses (either registered nurse [RN] or advanced practice registered nurses [APRN]), and only two did not include physicians (Lang et al., 2010; Rask et al., 2007); however, the specific number of participating physicians often was not reported. Four studies specifically listed doctorate of pharmacy (PharmD) participation, eight reported therapist participation, nine reported technician participation, and four reported social worker participation. Other reported participants included nutritionist, housekeeping, scheduler, physician assistant, unit secretary, chaplain, psychologist, and security officer. The accuracy of these counts is limited because some of these participants may have been included in a broad description such as "ancillary personnel," "support personnel," "OR team," "health care team," and "health care assistants." The number of patient and provider outcomes measured in each study also varied widely. For example, one study reported patient outcomes for only 21 patients (Helitzer et al., 2011), whereas another reported outcomes for 21,409 patients (Thompson et al., 2000a).

Setting

This review included studies reflecting a broad range of locales, including inpatient and outpatient settings. Interestingly, there were similar numbers of U.S. studies conducted in community hospitals and practices (14) and in academic health centers (15). The OR was the most commonly studied academic setting, accounting for six studies (Armour Forse et al., 2011; Bliss et al., 2012; Halverson et al., 2009; Nurok et al., 2011; Sax et al., 2009; Wolf et al., 2010). Acute care settings accounted for 10 of the 13 U.S. studies conducted in the community, while primary care clinics (including mental health) accounted for only 3 studies (Taylor et al., 2007; Thompson et al., 2000b; Young et al., 2005). The Veterans Health Administration hosted three large studies (Neily et al., 2010; Strasser et al., 2008; Young-Xu et al., 2011). Five international studies were included (Britain = three, Germany = one, Mexico = one). An unusual setting for reporting team training was U.S. combat operations in Iraq. Finally, one nursing home and one free-standing MRI facility were included.

Type of IPE Intervention

The type of IPE intervention varied widely. The two most cited interventions were Crew Resource Management (n = 9) and TeamSTEPPS (n = 6) (see Table A-2 in Annex A-1); however, these were almost always implemented in a modified format. Several other standardized programs were used (see Annex A-1), but in-house-designed programs were the most common type of IPE intervention. The descriptions of these programs varied from general and nonspecific to highly detailed. Several studies combined teamwork training with training focused on selected care outcomes, such as prevention of venous thromboembolism (Pingleton et al., 2013; Tapson et al., 2011) or best practices in diabetes management (Barceló et al., 2010; Janson et al., 2009; Taylor et al., 2007).

Overview of Findings

Learner teamwork competencies and communication skills were improved in most of the observational studies. Morbidity and mortality were directly measured in some of the larger studies, especially those focused on the OR (Armour Forse et al., 2011; Bliss et al., 2012; Neily et al., 2010; Young-Xu et al., 2011) and labor and delivery (Riley et al., 2011). One study looked at teamwork during resuscitations in the ICU and found significant improvements in survival (Knight et al., 2014). Care quality was improved in the majority of studies included in this review, most often reported as changes in practice processes, such as adherence to best practices, use of checklists, and participation in briefings. For most of these studies, team training was implemented as one part of a more comprehensive approach to practice changes (e.g., procedure manuals, mandatory OR briefings, checklists, new reporting systems). Improvements in specific patient care quality outcomes, such as HgbA1C, cholesterol, blood pressure, and mobility after stroke, were reported in four studies (Barceló et al., 2010; Janson et al., 2009; Strasser et al., 2008; Taylor et al., 2007). Patient safety outcomes were also improved in most studies as measured by decreases in adverse outcomes (Bliss et al., 2012; Mayer et al., 2011; Patterson et al., 2013; Pettker et al., 2009; Phipps et al., 2012; Pingleton et al., 2013; Riley et al., 2011) and error reporting (Hoffmann et al., 2014). A reduction in error rates was reported in two studies (Deering et al., 2011; Morey et al., 2002). Patient satisfaction was improved in two studies (Banki et al., 2013; Campbell et al., 2001) and unchanged in two others (Brown et al., 1999; Morey et al., 2002). Care efficiency improvements were measured in several studies (Banki et al., 2013; Capella et al., 2010; Wolf et al., 2010), and direct improvements in costs were reported in one study (Banki et al., 2013).

Overview of Methodologic Limitations

The following methodologic limitations were noted:

- for controlled studies, inability to control for differences between control and intervention study groups, lack of concealed allocation, inadequate blinding in the assessment of outcomes, evidence of selective outcome reporting, differences in the type and quality of the educational intervention, and difficult-to-measure endpoints;
- inadequate control for multiple other simultaneous practice changes that affect patient outcomes;
- lack of adequate timeline to document sustained changes in practice or patient outcomes;
- paucity of evidence for patient-centered changes in care;
- lack of studies addressing cost outcomes (business case);
- poor description of participants (how many, which disciplines);
- lack of clarity as to whether those trained together actually worked as a team in the practice setting;
- lack of evidence that teamwork training resulted in improved teamwork behaviors prior to assessment of clinical outcomes; and
- lack of adequate description of the type and quality of the IPE intervention as significant variables influencing outcomes.

DISCUSSION

The number of studies that link IPE with changes in practice and patient outcomes is growing. However, methodologic limitations continue to confound interpretation and generalization of the results.

While the RCT is considered the "gold standard" methodology for clinical studies, for educational research, they (like CBAs) suffer from less well-matched controls resulting from differences both within and among care delivery settings. Smaller studies are particularly vulnerable to the impact of differences among study groups. These barriers can be minimized to some degree by large-scale studies in which many clinician learners and practice settings can be randomized; however, differences among study sites likely remain, limiting meaningful comparisons in measured outcomes. Other methodological challenges related to participant allocation, investigator blinding, and variations in the quality of the IPE intervention cannot be completely avoided (Sullivan, 2011). As was stated in an Institute of Medicine (IOM) report on continuing medical education, "While controlled trial methods produce quantifiable end points, they do not fully explain whether outcomes occur as a result of participation in CE [continuing education], thus, a variety of research methods may be necessary" (IOM, 2010, p. 39).

Regardless of the study type, the implementation of other practice changes during the course of the study makes it difficult to ascribe documented changes in outcomes directly to the IPE intervention alone. One can argue that a combination of teamwork training and other practice changes would likely be even more effective in improving care (Weaver et al., 2014). Nevertheless, it is still important to better understand the independent and relative impact of teamwork training given the challenges inherent in scheduling and appropriately implementing effective IPE interventions.

The choice of outcome measures and measurement tools is a complex decision. Most of the studies in this review used retrieval of data from medical records to identify patient and practice outcome measures. While broad justifications are included in the background or introduction portions of these articles, few of the investigators make clear why particular outcome measures were chosen. At least three limitations should be considered when interpreting these data. First, studies using aggregate data collected from medical records pre- and postintervention are less likely to account for other changes in care unrelated to the IPE intervention than are studies in which specific cohorts of patients are carefully monitored and compared over time. Second, as described in the 2013 Cochrane review (Reeves et al., 2013), careful reading suggests that at least some studies engaged in selective reporting of outcomes, which limits complex interpretation of the effectiveness of the intervention. Finally, it is of concern that only four studies in this review focused on patient and family satisfaction. While objective measurement of practice and patient outcomes is essential, a patient-centered approach requires a more focused and nuanced tool for linking teamwork-based changes in care with the patient and family experience. Patients should not only be safe and well cared for, but should also feel safe and well cared for, and it is important to identify those teamwork factors that best promote that perception. Future research should focus on developing IPE interventions that teach patient-centered skills along with those skills needed to affect objective outcomes.

As with any education intervention, there is concern that the impact on knowledge, skills, and behavior will decay over time. All 11 of the long-term studies included in this review document a sustained impact on provider or patient outcomes, although the effects tended to decay over time. This is consistent with a 2007 comprehensive analysis of the effectiveness of continuing medical education (CME) in imparting knowledge and skills, changing attitudes and practice behavior, and improving clinical outcomes (Marinopoulos et al., 2007). While fewer than half of the studies in that analysis measured outcomes beyond 30 days postintervention, those that did found sustained changes in practice behaviors. Additional studies are needed to explore the best timing, content, format, and length of IPE interventions to provide the most sustained impact.

One challenge is that care-delivery in most institutions does not occur in the context of stable teams composed of professionals who train and work together in an intact group. Teams are most often ad hoc and may change on a weekly, daily, or even hourly basis for any given patient. With the exception of some of the operating room studies in this review, it is not clear whether the teams that trained together actually functioned as a team at the bedside. Although one meta-analysis suggests that improvements in team performance with team training are similar for intact and ad hoc teams (Salas et al., 2008), it may be that a team needs a "critical mass" of trained members in order to function effectively. Furthermore, while many of the studies provide the overall number of trainees and a list of partici-pating professions, few document whether the teams that participated in any specific training session actually represented an appropriate number of trainees from each profession. These limitations suggest that the demonstra-tion of improved teamwork skills in the actual clinical setting is an essential step before measuring practice or patient outcomes. While the Hawthorne effect is a consideration, there is evidence that observation in the clinical setting does not result in prolonged contamination of the data (Hohenhaus et al., 2008; Schnelle et al., 2006). Observation of actual changes in team behaviors provides stronger evidence for the link between team training and measureable changes in practice and patient outcomes (Morey and Salisbury, 2002).

It is interesting to note that few of the studies in this review gave in-depth consideration to the influence of IPE intervention implementation factors (timing, content, format, length, instructor and learner prepara-tion) on outcomes. Even when researchers used well-respected programs such as Crew Resource Management and TeamSTEPPS, the programs were frequently modified for logistical reasons. It is impossible to know how the modifications affected the outcomes; for that reason, the studies can-not be compared as if the same intervention were tested. The majority of investigators created IPE interventions of their own design. Many of the most effective IPE interventions in this review combined team training with "taskwork" training related to best practices for a specific patient population (e.g., diabetes patients). Salas and colleagues (2008) report that both teamwork and taskwork are effective in improving outcomes; however, the relative emphasis of each in the interventions in this study is not well described. IPE interventions that are created by local stakeholders to address institutional priorities have the advantage of eliciting increased participation by providers, integrating faculty development, and allowing for assessment of specific teamwork behaviors and competencies (Owen et al., 2012), but they often vary widely in scope, content, format, and dura-tion. There is a great deal of information available to inform the design and implementation of continuing IPE programs. Core principles that should be applied include ensuring adequate incorporation of effective theoretical foundations, adult learning principles, interprofessional learning objectives, and strategies for increased knowledge transfer and retention (IOM, 2013; Merriam and Leahy, 2005; Owen et al., 2014; Reeves and Hean, 2013). Yet for many of the studies in this review, it is not clear whether evidence-based principles were applied to the design and implementation of the IPE interventions. More guidance may be needed to help investigators choose the best approach.

Given the many methodologic limitations of these studies, outcome data must be interpreted carefully. Yet it is important to note that the majority of studies in this review found improvements in care processes, patient outcomes, or both. While the diversity of approaches and methodologic limitations make it difficult to draw clear conclusions with respect to best practices for linking IPE with patient and practice outcomes, this limited review suggests that the characteristics of those studies with the most significant improvements in outcomes include

- high learner participation rates or self-selection to intervention group,
- combination of IPE and goal-specific education (teamwork + taskwork),
- combination of IPE and other changes in practice processes,
- use of simulation and videotaping,
- repetition of IPE interventions with regular feedback to learners, and
- correlation of IPE intervention with observed and measurable changes in teamwork behaviors/skills.

While this review has attempted to describe the limitations of current research methodologies so that recommendations for future research can be made, it is important to recognize that many of the studies in this review represent high-quality groundbreaking research in a highly complex area of investigation. As stated in the 2010 IOM report, "In health care settings, it may remain difficult to measure dependent variables because linking participation in CE to changes in the practice setting is a complex process that cannot easily be tracked using current methods" (IOM, 2010, p. 35). In a recent synthesis of the team-training research literature, Weaver and colleagues (2014) note that research in this area is still plagued with limitations, including "small sample sizes, weak study design and limited detail regarding the team training curriculum or implementation strategy." When research limitations are compounded by the complexities of bringing together professionals from diverse backgrounds and perspectives, it is unsurprising that much work remains to be done.

AUTHORS' CONCLUSIONS

Based on this extensive review, it is the authors' opinion that key recommendations necessary for meaningful research linking IPE interventions with sustained changes in practice and patient outcomes include the following:

- Conduct large-scale controlled studies that minimize confounding variables; when this is not possible, consideration should be given to conducting well-designed ITS studies with careful monitoring of the study cohort to account for other variables that may impact outcomes.
- Use objective, relevant provider and patient outcome measures chosen prospectively, and report all results.
- Implement the IPE intervention at a defined time and adequately isolated from other practice changes.
- Collect pre- and postintervention data at multiple time points over several years.
- Include in patient outcome data an assessment of patient-centered team-based care.
- Observe and measure team behaviors in the actual practice setting before collecting practice or patient outcome data.
- Ensure that the IPE intervention is evidence- and competency-based, builds on sound theoretical underpinnings, is conducted by well-trained instructors, and is provided to the proper mix of learners.

REFERENCES

Armour Forse, R., J. D. Bramble, and R. McQuillan. 2011. Team training can improve operating room performance. *Surgery* 150(4):771-778.

Banki, F., K. Ochoa, M. E. Carrillo, S. S. Leake, A. L. Estrera, K. Khalil, and H. J. Safi. 2013. A surgical team with focus on staff education in a community hospital improves outcomes, costs and patient satisfaction. *American Journal of Surgery* 206(6):1007-1014; discussion 1014-1015.

Barceló, A., E. Cafiero, M. de Boer, A. E. Mesa, M. G. Lopez, R. A. Jimenez, A. L. Esqueda, J. A. Martinez, E. M. Holguin, M. Meiners, G. M. Bonfil, S. N. Ramirez, E. P. Flores, and S. Robles. 2010. Using collaborative learning to improve diabetes care and outcomes: The VIDA project. *Primary Care Diabetes* 4(3):145-153.

Bliss, L. A., C. B. Ross-Richardson, L. J. Sanzari, D. S. Shapiro, A. E. Lukianoff, B. A. Bernstein, and S. J. Ellner. 2012. Thirty-day outcomes support implementation of a surgical safety checklist. *Journal of the American College of Surgeons* 215(6):766-776.

Brown, J. B., M. Boles, J. P. Mullooly, and W. Levinson. 1999. Effect of clinician communication skills training on patient satisfaction. A randomized, controlled trial. *Annals of Internal Medicine* 131(11):822-829.

Campbell, J. C., J. H. Coben, E. McLoughlin, S. Dearwater, G. Nah, N. Glass, D. Lee, and N. Durborow. 2001. An evaluation of a system-change training model to improve emergency department response to battered women. *Academic Emergency Medicine* 8(2):131-138.

Capella, J., S. Smith, A. Philp, T. Putnam, C. Gilbert, W. Fry, E. Harvey, A. Wright, K. Henderson, and D. Baker. 2010. Teamwork training improves the clinical care of trauma patients. *Journal of Surgical Education* 67(6):439-443.

Deering, S., M. A. Rosen, V. Ludi, M. Munroe, A. Pocrnich, C. Laky, and P. G. Napolitano. 2011. On the front lines of patient safety: Implementation and evaluation of team training in Iraq. *Joint Commission Journal on Quality & Patient Safety* 37(8):350-356.

DeVita, M. A., J. Schaefer, J. Lutz, H. Wang, and T. Dongilli. 2005. Improving medical emergency team (MET) performance using a novel curriculum and a computerized human patient simulator. *Quality & Safety in Health Care* 14(5):326-331.

Halverson, A. L., J. L. Andersson, K. Anderson, J. Lombardo, C. S. Park, A. W. Rademaker, and D. W. Moorman. 2009. Surgical team training: The Northwestern Memorial Hospital experience. *Archives of Surgery* 144(2):107-112.

Hanbury, A., L. Wallace, and M. Clark. 2009. Use of a time series design to test effectiveness of a theory-based intervention targeting adherence of health professionals to a clinical guideline. *British Journal of Health Psychology* 14(Pt. 3):505-518.

Helitzer, D. L., M. Lanoue, B. Wilson, B. U. de Hernandez, T. Warner, and D. Roter. 2011. A randomized controlled trial of communication training with primary care providers to improve patient-centeredness and health risk communication. *Patient Education and Counseling* 82(1):21-29.

Hoffmann, B., V. Muller, J. Rochon, M. Gondan, B. Muller, Z. Albay, K. Weppler, M. Leifermann, C. Miessner, C. Guthlin, D. Parker, G. Hofinger, and F. M. Gerlach. 2014. Effects of a team-based assessment and intervention on patient safety culture in general practice: An open randomised controlled trial. *BMJ Quality and Safety* 23(1):35-46.

Hohenhaus, S. M., S. Powell, and R. Haskins. 2008. A practical approach to observation of the emergency care setting. *Journal of Emergency Nursing* 34(2):142-144.

IOM (Institute of Medicine). 2010. *Redesigning continuing education in the health professions.* Washington, DC: The National Academies Press.

IOM. 2013. *Interprofessional education for collaboration: Learning how to improve health from interprofessional models across the continuum of education to practice: Workshop summary.* Washington, DC: The National Academies Press.

Janson, S. L., M. Cooke, K. W. McGrath, L. A. Kroon, S. Robinson, and R. B. Baron. 2009. Improving chronic care of type 2 diabetes using teams of interprofessional learners. *Academic Medicine* 84(11):1540-1548.

Knight, L. J., J. M. Gabhart, K. S. Earnest, K. M. Leong, A. Anglemyer, and D. Franzon. 2014. Improving code team performance and survival outcomes: Implementation of pediatric resuscitation team training. *Critical Care Medicine* 42(2):243-251.

Lang, E. V., C. Ward, and E. Laser. 2010. Effect of team training on patients' ability to complete MRI examinations. *Academic Radiology* 17(1):18-23.

Marinopoulos, S. S., T. Dorman, N. Ratanawongsa, L. M. Wilson, B. H. Ashar, J. L. Magaziner, R. G. Miller, P. A. Thomas, G. P. Prokopowicz, R. Qayyum, and E. B. Bass. 2007. *Effectiveness of continuing medical education.* Evidence Report/Technology Assessment No. 149. Rockville, MD: Agency for Healthcare Research and Quality.

Mayer, C. M., L. Cluff, W. T. Lin, T. S. Willis, R. E. Stafford, C. Williams, R. Saunders, K. A. Short, N. Lenfestey, H. L. Kane, and J. B. Amoozegar. 2011. Evaluating efforts to optimize TeamSTEPPS implementation in surgical and pediatric intensive care units. *Joint Commission Journal on Quality and Patient Safety* 37(8):365-374.

Merriam, S. B., and B. Leahy. 2005. Learning transfer: A review of the research in adult education and training. *PAACE Journal of Lifelong Learning* 14:1-24.

Morey, J. C., and M. Salisbury. 2002. *Introducing teamwork training into healthcare organizations: Implementation issues and solutions.* Proceedings of the Human Factors and Ergonomics Society Annual Meeting, Baltimore, MD. Santa Monica, CA: Human Factors and Ergonomics Society. Pp. 2069-2073.

Morey, J. C., R. Simon, G. D. Jay, R. L. Wears, M. Salisbury, K. A. Dukes, and S. D. Berns. 2002. Error reduction and performance improvement in the emergency department through formal teamwork training: Evaluation results of the MedTeams project. *Health Services Research Journal* 37(6):1553-1581.

Neily, J., P. D. Mills, Y. Young-Xu, B. T. Carney, P. West, D. H. Berger, L. M. Mazzia, D. E. Paull, and J. P. Bagian. 2010. Association between implementation of a medical team training program and surgical mortality. *Journal of the American Medical Association* 304(15):1693-1700.

Nielsen, P. E., M. B. Goldman, S. Mann, D. E. Shapiro, R. G. Marcus, S. D. Pratt, P. Greenberg, P. McNamee, M. Salisbury, D. J. Birnbach, P. A. Gluck, M. D. Pearlman, H. King, D. N. Tornberg, and B. P. Sachs. 2007. Effects of teamwork training on adverse outcomes and process of care in labor and delivery: A randomized controlled trial. *Obstetrics & Gynecology* 109(1):48-55.

Nurok, M., L. A. Evans, S. Lipsitz, P. Satwicz, A. Kelly, and A. Frankel. 2011. The relationship of the emotional climate of work and threat to patient outcome in a high-volume thoracic surgery operating room team. *BMJ Quality and Safety* 20(3):237-242.

Owen, J. A., V. L. Brashers, C. Peterson, L. Blackhall, and J. Erickson. 2012. Collaborative care best practice models: A new educational paradigm for developing interprofessional educational (IPE) experiences. *Journal of Interprofessional Care* 26(2):153-155.

Owen, J. A., V. L. Brashers, K. E. Littlewood, E. Wright, R. M. Childress, and S. Thomas. 2014. Designing and evaluating an effective theory-based continuing interprofessional education program to improve sepsis care by enhancing healthcare team collaboration. *Journal of Interprofessional Care* 28(3):212-217.

Patterson, M. D., G. L. Geis, T. LeMaster, and R. L. Wears. 2013. Impact of multidisciplinary simulation-based training on patient safety in a paediatric emergency department. *BMJ Quality and Safety* 22(5):383-393.

Pettker, C. M., S. F. Thung, E. R. Norwitz, C. S. Buhimschi, C. A. Raab, J. A. Copel, E. Kuczynski, C. J. Lockwood, and E. F. Funai. 2009. Impact of a comprehensive patient safety strategy on obstetric adverse events. *American Journal of Obstetrics and Gynecology* 200(5):492.e1-492.e8.

Phipps, M. G., D. G. Lindquist, E. McConaughey, J. A. O'Brien, C. A. Raker, and M. J. Paglia. 2012. Outcomes from a labor and delivery team training program with simulation component. *American Journal of Obstetrics and Gynecology* 206(1):3-9.

Pingleton, S. K., E. Carlton, S. Wilkinson, J. Beasley, T. King, C. Wittkopp, M. Moncure, and T. Williamson. 2013. Reduction of venous thromboembolism (VTE) in hospitalized patients: Aligning continuing education with interprofessional team-based quality improvement in an academic medical center. *Academic Medicine* 88(10):1454-1459.

Rask, K., P. A. Parmelee, J. A. Taylor, D. Green, H. Brown, J. Hawley, L. Schild, H. S. Strothers III, and J. G. Ouslander. 2007. Implementation and evaluation of a nursing home fall management program. *Journal of the American Geriatric Society* 55(3):342-349.

Reeves, S., and S. Hean. 2013. Why we need theory to help us better understand the nature of interprofessional education, practice and care. *Journal of Interprofessional Care* 27(1):1-3.

Reeves, S., L. Perrier, J. Goldman, D. Freeth, and M. Zwarenstein. 2013. Interprofessional education: Effects on professional practice and healthcare outcomes (update). *Cochrane Database of Systematic Reviews* 3:CD002213.

Riley, W., S. Davis, K. Miller, H. Hansen, F. Sainfort, and R. Sweet. 2011. Didactic and simulation nontechnical skills team training to improve perinatal patient outcomes in a community hospital. *Joint Commission Journal on Quality and Patient Safety* 37(8):357-364.

Salas, E., D. DiazGranados, C. Klein, C. S. Burke, K. C. Stagl, G. F. Goodwin, and S. M. Halpin. 2008. Does team training improve team performance? A meta-analysis. *Human Factors: The Journal of the Human Factors and Ergonomics Society* 50(6):903-933.

Sax, H. C., P. Browne, R. J. Mayewski, R. J. Panzer, K. C. Hittner, R. L. Burke, and S. Coletta. 2009. Can aviation-based team training elicit sustainable behavioral change? *Archives of Surgery* 144(12):1133-1137.

Schnelle, J. F., J. G. Ouslander, and S. F. Simmons. 2006. Direct observations of nursing home care quality: Does care change when observed? *Journal of the American Medical Directors Association* 7(9):541-544.

Shaw, D. J., J. E. Davidson, R. I. Smilde, T. Sondoozi, and D. Agan. 2014. Multidisciplinary team training to enhance family communication in the ICU. *Critical Care Medicine* 42(2):265-271.

Steinemann, S., B. Berg, A. Skinner, A. DiTulio, K. Anzelon, K. Terada, C. Oliver, H. C. Ho, and C. Speck. 2011. In situ, multidisciplinary, simulation-based teamwork training improves early trauma care. *Journal of Surgical Education* 68(6):472-477.

Strasser, D. C., J. A. Falconer, A. B. Stevens, J. M. Uomoto, J. Herrin, S. E. Bowen, and A. B. Burridge. 2008. Team training and stroke rehabilitation outcomes: A cluster randomized trial. *Archives of Physical Medicine & Rehabilitation* 89(1):10-15.

Sullivan, G. M. 2011. Getting off the "gold standard": Randomized controlled trials and education research. *Journal of Graduate Medical Education* 3(3):285-289.

Tapson, V. F., R. B. Karcher, and R. Weeks. 2011. Crew resource management and VTE prophylaxis in surgery: A quality improvement initiative. *American Journal of Medical Quality* 26(6):423-432.

Taylor, C. R., J. T. Hepworth, P. I. Buerhaus, R. Dittus, and T. Speroff. 2007. Effect of crew resource management on diabetes care and patient outcomes in an inner-city primary care clinic. *Quality & Safety in Health Care* 16(4):244-247.

Theilen, U., P. Leonard, P. Jones, R. Ardill, J. Weitz, D. Agrawal, and D. Simpson. 2013. Regular in situ simulation training of paediatric medical emergency team improves hospital response to deteriorating patients. *Resuscitation* 84(2):218-222.

Thompson, C., A. L. Kinmonth, L. Stevens, R. C. Peveler, A. Stevens, K. J. Ostler, R. M. Pickering, N. G. Baker, A. Henson, J. Preece, D. Cooper, and M. J. Campbell. 2000a. Effects of a clinical-practice guideline and practice-based education on detection and outcome of depression in primary care: Hampshire depression project randomised controlled trial. *Lancet* 355(9199):185-191.

Thompson, R. S., F. P. Rivara, D. C. Thompson, W. E. Barlow, N. K. Sugg, R. D. Maiuro, and D. M. Rubanowice. 2000b. Identification and management of domestic violence: A randomized trial. *American Journal of Preventive Medicine* 19(4):253-263.

Weaver, S. J., M. A. Rosen, D. DiazGranados, E. H. Lazzara, R. Lyons, E. Salas, S. A. Knych, M. McKeever, L. Adler, M. Barker, and H. B. King. 2010. Does teamwork improve performance in the operating room? A multilevel evaluation. *Joint Commission Journal on Quality and Patient Safety* 36(3):133-142.

Weaver, S. J., S. M. Dy, and M. A. Rosen. 2014. Team-training in healthcare: A narrative synthesis of the literature. *BMJ Quality and Safety* 23(5):359-372.

Wolf, F. A., L. W. Way, and L. Stewart. 2010. The efficacy of medical team training: Improved team performance and decreased operating room delays: A detailed analysis of 4863 cases. *Annals of Surgery* 252(3):477-483.

Young, A. S., M. Chinman, S. L. Forquer, E. L. Knight, H. Vogel, A. Miller, M. Rowe, and J. Mintz. 2005. Use of a consumer-led intervention to improve provider competencies. *Psychiatric Services* 56(8):967-975.

Young-Xu, Y., J. Neily, P. D. Mills, B. T. Carney, P. West, D. H. Berger, L. M. Mazzia, D. E. Paull, and J. P. Bagian. 2011. Association between implementation of a medical team training program and surgical morbidity. *Archives of Surgery* 146(12):1368-1373.

ANNEX A-1

TABLE A-2 Measuring the Impact of IPE on Collaborative Practice and Patient Outcomes: Detailed Data Table

Study	Score	Outcome Measures	Measurement Tool	Type of Study	Sample Size
Brown et al., 1999	IA	Patient satisfaction; patient assessment of clinician's communication skills (Art of Medicine anonymous survey)	Art of Medicine survey that was mailed to patients 19 days postvisit	Randomized controlled trial (RCT)	69 providers consisting of MDs, nurse practitioners (NPs), physician assistants (PAs), optometrists (MDs 75 percent of sample size)
Campbell et al., 2001	IB	Rates of reported intimate partner violence (IPV), patient satisfaction. Staff knowledge and attitudes, "culture of the ED" (met Joint Commission on Accreditation of Hospitals [JCAH] protocols, IPV materials in emergency room [ER], regular staff training), patient satisfaction, identification rates of battered women	1. Clinical documentation 2. Observable measures of "culture" 3. Staff attitudinal study (not validated)	RCT	12 hospitals, 649 clinicians; MDs, RNs, social workers (SWs), administrators trained; only MDs and RNs studied; 600 patients

Setting	Intervention (description)	Findings	Comments (EKP, JKM, VLB)
Community general acute	Communication skills training, which consisted of an initial 4-hour workshop, 2 hours homework, and a 4-hour follow-up workshop. Viewed videotapes of own practice behaviors.	Participants self-reported moderate improvement in communication skills, but patient satisfaction scores did not improve. Mean score improved more in control than in intervention group.	Training focused on communication with patients, not on teamwork skills per se, and changes in communication skills not related to teamwork (provider to patient only). Needed control group trained with same information in uniprofessional groups.
Community emergency department	Teams participated in a 2-day didactic information and team planning intervention, addressing systems change and coalition building, provider attitudes, and skill building. Teams were asked to meet before and after training to develop and implement an action plan.	Experimental emergency departments (EDs) were significantly higher than the control EDs on staff knowledge and attitudes, the summary score of culture criteria, and patient satisfaction. No significant differences were found between self-reported battered women and clinically identified abused women in experimental versus control hospitals.	Only one hospital sent complete team measurement: "Culture of ED" system-change indicator (not validated); not all hospitals sent a full complement of team members. Time between training and implementation of routine screening averaged 10 months.

continued

TABLE A-2 Continued

Study	Score	Outcome Measures	Measurement Tool	Type of Study	Sample Size
Helitzer et al., 2011	IA	Provider-with-patient communication proficiency in simulated and actual patient visits using Roter Interaction Analysis System (RIAS) coding of patient-centeredness communication skills plus coding of 21 additional communication proficiencies	Roter Interaction Analysis System	RCT	26 clinicians = 22 MDs, 2 PAs, 2 NPs; 21 patient visits
Hoffmann et al., 2014	IB	Primary outcome was indicator error management; secondary outcomes were indicators of patient safety culture, data on patient safety climate and volume and quality of incident reporting	Assessment of quality indicators and safety incident reporting	RCT	60 practices, randomized to one of two groups = MDs, health care assistants

Setting	Intervention (description)	Findings	Comments (EKP, JKM, VLB)
Academic primary care	Full-day training, individualized feedback on videotaped interactions with simulated patients, and optional workshops to reinforce strategies for engaging patients.	Intervention providers significantly improved in patient-centeredness communication and communication proficiencies immediately post-training and at two follow-up visits.	Randomized and controlled. Link between training and skills using simulation established prior to measuring actual practice setting. Outcomes measured longitudinally all the way to 2 years. Note: Small sample size, but even with this size, significant differences were found. Question whether training together had any additional impact compared with training separately.
German general practices	Team session describing the intervention and instructing on the instrument (FraTrix), then three facilitated team sessions over 9 months using the instrument.	No significant differences at 12 months between groups in error management, 11 patient safety culture indicators, and safety climate scales. Intervention practices showed better reporting of patient safety incidents (significant increase in the number and quality of incident reports).	Significant participation, with entire team attending >90 percent of training sessions in intervention group. But study groups were self-selected; intervention group might have already been more committed to change. Not clear what a "health care assistant" is.

continued

TABLE A-2 Continued

Study	Score	Outcome Measures	Measurement Tool	Type of Study	Sample Size
Nielson et al., 2007	IB	Patient outcomes: proportion of deliveries at ≥20 weeks in which ≥1 adverse maternal or neonatal outcomes occurred; process measures: time from registration to provider assessment, registration to maternal fetal assessment, registration to induction, group B streptococci antibiotic order to first dose, epidural request to initiation, scheduled C-section start time to incision, immediate C-section decision to incision, urgent C-section decision to incision, registration to delivery nullipara, registration to delivery multipara, delivery to end of care in labor and delivery (L&D)	Clinical documentation + 11 clinical process measures	Cluster RCT	15 hospitals of various types, 1,307 personnel = MDs, RNs; 28,536 birth outcomes

Setting	Intervention (description)	Findings	Comments (EKP, JKM, VLB)
Community labor and delivery (military and civilian)	One 4-hour standardized teamwork training. Curriculum based on crew resource management. Added on call contingency to respond to obstetric (OB) emergencies (MedTeams Labor & Delivery Team Coordination Course). Clinical staff attended 3-day instructor training session; trainers returned to hospitals to conduct onsite training sessions for staff. Also, a contingency team (experienced MDs and RNs) was trained to respond in a coordinated way to OB emergencies, drawing on additional resources as necessary.	No statistically significant differences between groups in clinical adverse events. Only time from decision to perform immediate C-section to incision was significantly ($P = 0.03$) lower in intervention group.	Large study. Lacked sufficient description of trainees. Question whether duration of intervention was adequate to change so many outcomes.

continued

TABLE A-2 Continued

Study	Score	Outcome Measures	Measurement Tool	Type of Study	Sample Size
Nurok et al., 2011	IB	Threat to patient outcomes	Observation using a standardized observation tool that describes interprofessional (IP) behaviors (briefing, debriefing, Situation Background Assessment Recommendation [SBAR], knowledge sharing, closed-loop communication, conflict resolution, debriefing, and threats to patient outcomes)	RCT	Unclear number of providers trained = MDs, RNs, technicians; 105 surgical cases observed
Riley et al., 2011	IB	Ten weighted perinatal outcome measures	Weighted Adverse Outcomes Scores (WAOS) for obstetric care—average adverse event score per delivery weighted for severity of events	Cluster RCT	3 hospitals; 135 clinicians = MDs, RNs, certified registered nurse assistants (CRNAs), PAs; approximately 1,500 deliveries

Setting	Intervention (description)	Findings	Comments (EKP, JKM, VLB)
Academic operating room	Training consisted of two 90-minute multidisciplinary team-skills training sessions.	Measures of teamwork described as "emotional climate" correlated with decreased threats to patient outcomes in the sterile surgical field environment.	Validated own observational tools and established interrater reliability. Specifics of "sustaining" time period not well described. The behaviors tended to diminish over time. There are a number of shortcomings, but the authors have done an excellent job of outlining the limitations.
Community labor and delivery	One hospital served as a control; a second hospital received the TeamSTEPPS didactic training program; a third hospital received the TeamSTEPPS didactic training program with in situ simulation training.	A statistically significant improvement in perinatal morbidity using the TeamSTEPPS with simulation training as compared with control; no statistical difference in TeamSTEPPS didactic only and control.	Methodology not clear on who was trained and how. Multiple data points reported over time period, but only aggregated results for significance factor. Would have been interesting to measure behaviors in simulated setting pre- and post-intervention to tease out how one TeamSTEPPS approach impacted competencies versus the other.

continued

TABLE A-2 Continued

Study	Score	Outcome Measures	Measurement Tool	Type of Study	Sample Size
Strasser et al., 2008	IB	Patient functional improvement as measured by three patient outcomes: (1) change in motor items, (2) community discharge, and (3) length of stay (LOS)	The FIM (Functional Independence Measure) instrument was used to measure changes in motor items	Cluster RCT	227 clinicians in 15 intervention teams and 237 clinicians in 16 control teams = MDs, RNs, occupational therapists (OTs), speech-language pathologists (SLPs), and SWs; 487 stroke patients

Setting	Intervention (description)	Findings	Comments (EKP, JKM, VLB)
Veterans Health Administration (VHA)	Six months of training over three phases on team dynamics, problem solving, use of feedback data, action plans for process improvement. Followed by workshop to create written action plans; third phase at months 3-6. Telephone and videoconference consultation. Team leaders received summaries of team's performance and suggestions on how to use the data.	For both stroke patients and all patients, there was a significant difference in improvement of functional outcomes between intervention and control groups. There were no significant difference in LOS or rates of community discharge.	Large study, randomized, clear outcome measurement related directly to the IPE intervention, robust training.

continued

TABLE A-2 Continued

Study	Score	Outcome Measures	Measurement Tool	Type of Study	Sample Size
Thompson et al., 2000a	IA	Practice: physician recognition of depression patients: proportion of patients with clinical improvement in depression	Validated Hospital Anxiety and Depression (HAD) Scale	RCT	60 practices and 21,409 patients/59 primary care practices (29/30); MDs, RNs

Setting	Intervention (description)	Findings	Comments (EKP, JKM, VLB)
Britain primary care	Seminars (4 hours). Used videotapes to demonstrate skills, small-group discussion of cases, and role play. Educators remained available to practices for ~9 months after seminars for additional information and help. Each participant completed a questionnaire after the seminars, and a video recording of one seminar was rated by independent experts. Teaching materials also rated.	Sensitivity of physicians to depressive symptoms was no different between intervention and control groups. Outcomes of depressed patients as a whole at 6 weeks or 6 months after assessment did not significantly improve.	Quality of training sessions not clearly described. Was the training about recognizing depression, or was there an element of teamwork training? Practice outcome measurement related only to physicians, not clear if anyone else had a role in affecting patient outcomes. Needs control group in which only physicians trained.

continued

TABLE A-2 Continued

Study	Score	Outcome Measures	Measurement Tool	Type of Study	Sample Size
Thompson et al., 2000b	IB	<u>Baseline and 9 months</u>: Provider knowledge, attitudes, and beliefs; <u>process</u>: recorded rates of questioning for domestic violence (DV); assessment of management plans for victims	Validated provider survey and clinical record review	RCT	5 clinics (exp. 2, control 3); 179 clinicians = MDs, NPs, PAs, RNs, LPNs, medical assistants (MAs)

Setting	Intervention (description)	Findings	Comments (EKP, JKM, VLB)
Community primary care	One-year intervention composed of two half-day training sessions, extra training for leaders, bimonthly newsletter, clinic educational rounds, system support (posters, cue cards, questionnaires), and feedback of results.	Four of the six provider survey domain scores improved from baseline to 9 months in intervention group. Improvements in three of these four domains remained significant at 21-23 months. At 9 months, intervention group saw improvement in awareness of DV guidelines and on rating of guidelines as useful, beliefs of not knowing how to ask, and not knowing what to do. Overall asking about DV was fourfold greater after intervention than in control clinics. Quality of patient management judged good or excellent at pre- and postintervention.	Unclear whether "team training" actually focused on teamwork rather than specific practice process changes (many other changes over the year of the study in addition to team training). Strength in reporting both objective case findings consistent with subjective outcome measures.

continued

TABLE A-2 Continued

Study	Score	Outcome Measures	Measurement Tool	Type of Study	Sample Size
Barceló et al., 2010	IIB	Patient: meeting quality improvement goals in A1C, cholesterol, blood pressure (BP), foot exam, eye exam, three or more treatment goals; Practice: organization of care, community linkages, self-management support, delivery system design, decision support, information system	Clinical database and Assessment of Chronic Illness Care evaluation	Controlled before-and-after (CBA)	307 patients; 43 primary care teams; MDs, RNs, nutritionist, psychologists (not random but rather specifically selected for willingness, communication, collaboration)

Setting	Intervention (description)	Findings	Comments (EKP, JKM, VLB)
Mexico public health centers	Three learning sessions using breakthrough series (BTS) methodology; includes strategies to improve quality of diabetes care: patient education program, training in foot care, and training for primary care personnel in diabetes management.	Proportion of patients achieving A1C <7 percent increased significantly among intervention group compared with usual care and for low total cholesterol. Proportion of patients receiving foot and eye exams also showed positive results among intervention group. Overall, the proportion of patients who achieved ≥3 quality improvement goals increased significantly among intervention group, while among usual care it decreased but not significantly.	While 81 percent of patients in intervention group participated, only 32 percent participated in usual care group. Discussion groups in intervention arm selected on personality not random assignment. Differences between patients in intervention and control groups may have skewed results. Centers were not standardized in intervention delivery (some centers focused on enhanced psychological support, increased physical activity, and improvement in the patient–provider relationship, but not all).

continued

TABLE A-2 Continued

Study	Score	Outcome Measures	Measurement Tool	Type of Study	Sample Size
Janson et al., 2009	IIB	Clinical assessments and processes of care: complete (A1C, low-density lipoprotein [LDL], BP, urine microalbumin, smoking assessment, foot exams)	Clinical database	CBA	384 patients: 148 learners = medical residents, NP students, pharmacy students; 28 residents were control group

Setting	Intervention (description)	Findings	Comments (EKP, JKM, VLB)
Academic primary care	Chronic illness curriculum simultaneous quality improvement (QI) projects based on Improving Chronic Illness Care (ICIC) model delivered by interprofessional faculty. Presentation topic on aspects of diabetes mellitus (DM) care. Didactic presentations, clinical discussions, and clinic visits with patients. Interprofessional team care provided by primary care internal medicine residents, nurse practitioner students, and pharmacy students.	Intervention patients received significantly more assessments of glycosylated hemoglobin, LDL, BP, microalbuminuria, and smoking status, and foot exams. Intervention patients had significantly more planned general medicine visits than control patients. Learners in intervention group had a significant increase in all measured components of ICIC model. Interprofessional learners rated themselves significantly higher on measures of accomplishment, preparation, and success for chronic care.	Many simultaneous interventions; difficult to determine whether any change is due specifically to IPE intervention.

continued

TABLE A-2 Continued

Study	Score	Outcome Measures	Measurement Tool	Type of Study	Sample Size
Morey et al., 2002	IIA	Team behavior, ED performance, and attitudes and opinions	(1) Team behaviors using Team Dimension Rating form, (2) National Aeronautics and Space Administration (NASA) task load index, (3) ED Staff Attitude and Opinion Survey, and (4) Patient Satisfaction Survey	CBA	6 EDs in the experimental group (684 clinicians) and 3 EDs in the control group (374 clinicians); 50 observed team interactions; MDs, RNs, technicians
Rask et al., 2007	IIB	Detailed process-of-care documentation, number of falls, use of restraints	24-item process-of-care audit tool and clinical database	CBA	42 nursing homes/19 intervention, 23 control; RNs, OTs, certified nursing assistants (CNAs), maintenance staff

Setting	Intervention (description)	Findings	Comments (EKP, JKM, VLB)
Community emergency department	Team training curriculum (Emergency Team Coordination Course [ETCC]). Eight hours of lecture and discussion reflecting five team dimensions. Also the ED teamwork reorganization followed the intervention. Training was developed by experts, behavioral scientists, and hospital staff.	Teamwork and quality of team behaviors improved significantly in the experimental group. No significant difference in subjective workload. Clinical error rate significantly declined in experimental group. ED staff attitudes toward teamwork and assessments of institutional support increased significantly in the experimental group. Patient satisfaction went up in experimental group and down in control group, but neither was significant.	Large study, well controlled. Team Dimensions Rating Form not validated for health care teams. Did follow outcomes out to 9 months. Blended staff and patient outcomes tools—items taken from several sources.
Nursing homes	Full-day workshop covering core program components and a second workshop 1 month later to address support modules and challenges. Also, manual and notebook with details of program implementation, videotape for training, and brochures for unit staff.	All 21 care process chart audits showed improvement between baseline and follow-up in intervention group; most were statistically significant. Trend in fall rates was not significant for intervention homes. Restraint use dropped across all homes at a significant rate.	Clear outcome measures and detailed audit tool. Documented results extended out many months. Makes strong case for direct link between training and improvements in outcomes.

continued

TABLE A-2 Continued

Study	Score	Outcome Measures	Measurement Tool	Type of Study	Sample Size
Weaver et al., 2010	IIB	(1) Trainee reactions, (2) trainee learning, (3) observed collaborative behaviors, and (4) results (degree to which teamwork behaviors enacted on the job produce safety-quality)	(1) Hospital survey on patient safety culture; (2) operating room management attitudes questionnaire; (3) Medical Performance Assessment tool for Communication & Teamwork (MedPACT)	CBA using historical controls but also contemporaneous control group with checklist only	55 clinicians; MDs, RNs, Techs, PAs, CRNAs

Setting	Intervention (description)	Findings	Comments (EKP, JKM, VLB)
Community general acute	TeamSTEPPS (core competencies-communication, leadership, mutual support, situation monitoring). Four-hour didactic session, including interactive role playing.	The trained group (TeamSTEPPS) demonstrated significant increases in the quantity and quality of presurgical procedure briefings and the use of quality teamwork behaviors during cases. Increases were also found in perceptions of patient safety culture and teamwork attitudes.	Validated own observational assessment tool of teamwork behaviors and practice processes. No patient outcomes.

continued

TABLE A-2 Continued

Study	Score	Outcome Measures	Measurement Tool	Type of Study	Sample Size
Young et al., 2005	IIB	Clinician competencies using Competency Assessment Instrument (CAI) treatment processes through qualitative interview; general competencies, assessment and treatment competencies, rehabilitation competencies, skill advocacy, overall competency, recovery orientation	Competency Assessment Instrument	CBA	269 clinicians/5 sites (1 in each state was the intervention site); therapists, RNs, case managers, MDs, administrators
Hanbury et al., 2009	IIB	Adherence to national suicide prevention guideline for community mental health professionals	Surveys and clinical record audit	Interrupted time series (ITS)	49 attended, 21 completed questionnaire; did not describe how many chart audits; "all community health professionals," RNs and MDs

Setting	Intervention (description)	Findings	Comments (EKP, JKM, VLB)
Community primary care	Education, clinician–client dialogues, technical assistance, support of self-help. Clinicians—scientific presentation on self-help, structured dialogues, rehabilitation readiness, strategies for independence, professional skills supporting self-help, detailing. Consumers—technical assistance, 1-day at site including research presentation, structured questions, and small-group discussion. Consumer leaders identified. Fund for logistical support.	Intervention group's scores on 10 competencies improved significantly compared with the control group. Competency regarding stigma worsened equally and significantly in both groups. No dose–response relationship for medication management. At 1 year, interviews showed intervention sites were providing more recovery-oriented services than control sites. Clinicians at intervention sites reported more support from management for implementing new rehabilitation services.	High clinician turnover; only 72 percent completed follow-up interview. Strength was focus on patient-centered outcomes rather than only clinician-centric processes.
Britain primary care	Educational session in three components about guideline, group discussions about beliefs, and group work on two real-life vignettes developed in house.	No impact on guideline adherence related to study intervention.	Developed and validated own tool. Large differences between control and intervention groups at outset. Unclear who was surveyed, who was audited. No description of the size or makeup of the training groups or whether teamwork was part of the learning objectives. Results impacted by outside events (publication of national guidelines).

continued

TABLE A-2 Continued

Study	Score	Outcome Measures	Measurement Tool	Type of Study	Sample Size
Pettker et al., 2009	IIB	Adverse Outcomes Index—number of deliveries with adverse events; rates of cesarean delivery, episiotomies, and shoulder dystocia	Clinical database	ITS	13,622 deliveries; 289 clinicians trained; MDs, RNs, "ancillary staff"
Taylor et al., 2007	IIB	Both process and patient outcome measures. Quarterly A1C (<7 percent), BP (<130/80), LDL (<100 mg/dl), urine microalbumin (<30/24), lower extremity amputation prevention (LEAP) foot checks	Clinical database and clinical observations	ITS	619 patients, 15 providers = advanced practice registered nurses (APRNs), "support staff"; administrators
Armour Forse et al., 2011	IIB	OR first case starts; Surgical Quality Improvement Program (SQIP = antibiotic administration, venous thromboembolism [VTE] prophylaxis, beta blocker administration, patient satisfaction); National SQIP (NSQIP) surgical mortality and morbidity	Hospital (OR starts) and public reported data (SQIP and NSQIP from American College of Surgeons)	Before-and-after (BA)	No N given for providers or patients; MDs, RNs, technicians

Setting	Intervention (description)	Findings	Comments (EKP, JKM, VLB)
Academic labor and delivery	Crew resource management (CRM).	Adverse Outcomes Index declined significantly, but many other initiatives started simultaneously so not clear if team training was a significant component.	Well-documented large study with impressive results over a relatively long time period. But numerous interventions; not clear whether team training alone played a significant role.
Community primary care	CRM—task redistribution, communication, decision (checklist) development using clinical guidelines.	Significant impact on three care processes and three patient outcomes.	Strength in ITS approach, which detected trends that would not have been observable with simple BA study. Team training included development of practice process checklists, so not clear if the training itself played a significant role.
Academic operating room	TeamSTEPPS.	Significant improvements in antibiotic administration, VTE prophylaxis, and beta blocker administration; surgical morbidity; and surgical mortality.	Strength in measuring six patient outcomes over 5-year period. Study issues: MDs were trained using an abbreviated program; full team was not trained together. NSQIP data show short-term improvement with long-term regression. Mortality has also returned to pretraining levels, and morbidity and complications increased after an initial decrease.

continued

TABLE A-2 Continued

Study	Score	Outcome Measures	Measurement Tool	Type of Study	Sample Size
Banki et al., 2013	IIB	Operative time and operating room (OR) costs; LOS and hospital room costs, patient satisfaction	Clinical database; Press Ganey tool, discharge instructions	BA	59 clinicians, 268 procedures: 193 before, 165 after; RNs, respiratory therapists (RTs), physical therapists (PTs), nutritionists, techs, assistants, MDs
Bliss et al., 2012	IIB	Qualitative: communication, decision making, equipment availability, equipment malfunction, disruptive behavior, process/ flow, sterility; Quantitative: completion of individual checklist items, 30-day morbidity (adverse events)	NSQIP tool used by a trained observer + expert review of clinical database	BA	2,079 historical controls, 246 cases without list, 73 cases with checklist use; type of clinicians and sample size not specified, but discussion suggests RNs and MDs participated

Setting	Intervention (description)	Findings	Comments (EKP, JKM, VLB)
Community operating room	Monthly teaching sessions with staff about decreasing time and costs, LOS, and room costs and improving patient satisfaction. Monthly multidisciplinary conferences, weekly meeting with team leaders, and daily patient rounds by surgeon and nurses.	Significant reductions in median operating time, LOS, OR costs, hospital room costs. There were significant improvements in communication with nurses, pain management, and communication about medicines.	The intervention simultaneously included many process changes and much special attention to the patients who were selected (private rooms, patient instructions, constant monitoring, consistent staff who were specially trained, low patient/nurse ratio), so it is difficult to demonstrate that the education intervention was the cause of any outcomes.
Academic operating room	Three 60-minute team training sessions focused on communication and orienting participants to the use of comprehensive surgical checklist.	Comparison of 30-day morbidity demonstrated significant reduction in overall adverse event rates from cases with only team training, and in cases with checklist use. Lack of confirmation of patient identity and failure to address procedure and procedure site were both significantly associated with higher occurrences of deep surgical site infections. Cases without documentation of the introduction of all team members were significantly more likely to include major morbidity and infectious events.	Prospective cohort design with historical controls. Large study, training provided to all OR personnel and compared with historical controls. Differences with historical controls impressive with training alone. Adding checklist improved outcomes further. Because the control for the team training was only historical, cannot be sure it was the training that caused the change, but appreciate separating out data related to training alone versus training plus checklist.

continued

TABLE A-2 Continued

Study	Score	Outcome Measures	Measurement Tool	Type of Study	Sample Size
Capella et al., 2010	IIC	Observed behaviors in the OR (Trauma Team Performance Observation Tool [TPOT]); time from arrival to computed tomography (CT), intubation, OR, and/or Sonography; time in ED; hospital LOS; intensive care unit (ICU) LOS; complications; mortality	TPOT (leadership, situation monitoring, mutual support, communication; hospital trauma registry	BA	114 providers; 73 resuscitations; surgery residents, MDs, nurses
Deering et al., 2011	IIB	Safety incidents, including medication and transfusion errors, communication-related errors, needlestick incidents	Safety incident reports	BA	>3,000 trained, but not clear how many were at the one center where outcomes were measured; MDs and RNs

Setting	Intervention (description)	Findings	Comments (EKP, JKM, VLB)
Academic emergency department	TeamSTEPPS didactic plus simulation. Didactic given to residents and attending trauma surgeons. Simulation with nurses as well.	Significant improvements in all parameters of TPOT; decreased time from arrival to CT, intubation, and OR. But no improvements in patient outcomes such as LOS, complication rate, or mortality rate.	Both self-perceived and patient outcome improvements after training. One institution only. Three-month sampling following intervention, during which time staff knew they were being evaluated. Convenience sample of resuscitations observed. Workers worked faster, but patient outcomes were not significantly different between the groups. Would have strengthened study if increased efficiency were linked to decreased costs.
Combat theater of operations, Baghdad	TeamSTEPPS modified (no simulation).	Significant decreases in rates of communication-related errors, medication and transfusion errors, and needlestick incidents.	Large number of trainees, but safety reports reviewed at only one center. Unusual setting—not generalizable Only a few were trained fully from each group. Training occurred in many different ways. Items were added to the data collection form and included steps that the staff were expected to go through during debrief. Did the intervention or the change in form account for the changes in behavior?

continued

TABLE A-2 Continued

Study	Score	Outcome Measures	Measurement Tool	Type of Study	Sample Size
Halverson et al., 2009	IIB	Preoperative briefing rates and components; observation of OR team performance; hospital metrics: rates of wrong side or site events or close calls, timely antibiotic administration; efficiency metrics: rate of on-time case starts and turnover time between cases	Hospital-based QI personnel OR observations (no checklist given but some items mentioned in text) and hospital metrics data	BA	1,150 trainees, 39 procedures; 156 completed post survey about perceptions of teamwork and usefulness of briefings
Knight et al., 2014	IIB	Primary outcome: Post-cardiopulmonary arrest survival to discharge; Secondary: (1) change in neurologic morbidity from admission to discharge, (2) improvement in pediatric code team performance	Review of CPR (cardio-pulmonary resuscitation) records for guideline adherence, clinical database	BA	"90% of core code team members" = MDs, RNs, RTs, PharmDs, SWs (no N given); 183 events preintervention (124 patients) and 65 events postintervention (46 patients)

Setting	Intervention (description)	Findings	Comments (EKP, JKM, VLB)
Academic operating room	Their own team-training curriculum, never published. Train the trainer model well described.	Better compliance with debriefings. No other changes other than perceptual.	Large study, strength in observing practice process changes before and then with measurement of patient outcomes. Impact of training on debriefings declined with time (6 months), and it is difficult to draw conclusions about the lack of impact on patient outcomes since compliance with debriefings does not describe the quality of those interactions or the presence of true teamwork.
Academic intensive care unit	Composite Resuscitation Team Training over 6-month period. Monthly videotaped in situ simulations—16 simulations were videotaped, and participants were debriefed. New training included new types of participants (professions) and additional training programs.	Intervention group patients statistically more likely to survive than control group; there was no significant change in neurologic morbidity. Intervention group participants statistically more likely to adhere to resuscitation standard operating procedure.	Historical control averaged over 4 years of data, Training of code team occurred during the 18-month intervention period—strength related to in situ simulation training. Training reinforced monthly; however, unclear if the original cohort ("90 percent") were retrained or only some of them. Outcomes data averaged over intervention period, so not clear whether skills increased or decreased over duration of the study, and no measurements reported for after training period ended.

continued

TABLE A-2 Continued

Study	Score	Outcome Measures	Measurement Tool	Type of Study	Sample Size
Lang et al., 2010	IIC	Patient completion of magnetic resonance imaging (MRI)	Department records	BA	N not provided; RNs, technologists, receptionists, schedulers
Mayer et al., 2011	IIB	Observed team behaviors; time to extracorporeal membrane oxygenation (ECMO); duration of adult surgery rapid response events; rate of nosocomial infections	National Database of Nursing Quality Indicators (NDNQI®); Teamwork Evaluation of Non-Technical Skills (TENTS) observation tool (communication, leadership, situation monitoring, mutual support); clinical timing data; clinical infection data	BA	For observed team behaviors, 56 teams before intervention, 38 at 1 month, 47 at 6 months, and 54 at 12 months; number of patients less clear; MDs, RNs, RTs

Setting	Intervention (description)	Findings	Comments (EKP, JKM, VLB)
Free-standing MRI facility	Team training in rapport, communication with patients, and self-hypnosis for patients.	Significant reduction in number of patients who could not complete their MRI.	One facility, intervention not well described, sample not well described, but included because of the unusual and important setting. Because an announcement was made that the practice was being dissolved, it is likely that numbers went down considerably. Does this matter? Are the teams "different" in important ways in the later stages of the study because of the announcement? With two different interventions, it is unclear if either one is responsible for the change in completion rates.
Academic intensive care unit	"Customized" TeamSTEPPS; TeamSTEPPS was modified, with reduction in amount of time trained.	Significant reduction in time to ECMO; Registered Respiratory Therapist (RRT) response time was not affected; however, there was an increased length of RRT events; percent infections lower than preintervention upper control limit.	Well-described intervention, but other changes in organizational processes likely affected outcomes, so that direct link with IPE difficult to make. Data reported at multiple timepoints; however, some selective reporting of data, and most outcomes averaged pre and post. This study found improvements, but saw a drift back to baseline rates.

continued

TABLE A-2 Continued

Study	Score	Outcome Measures	Measurement Tool	Type of Study	Sample Size
Neily et al., 2010	IIB	Surgical mortality	Clinical database	BA	108 facilities; MDs, RNs, technicians

Setting	Intervention (description)	Findings	Comments (EKP, JKM, VLB)
VHA	Medical Team Training (MTT) program based on CRM.	Significant reduction in surgical mortality.	Very large study; retrospective; contemporaneous control group improves study. CRM + numerous other interventions makes determining impact of IPE on outcomes difficult. The mortality rates at baseline were higher in intervention hospitals and the same as in untrained hospitals at the end of the study. Was their greater reduction due to regression to the mean of all hospitals? Interviews conducted only in training facilities. Staff "reported" improved communication, awareness, and teamwork. MTT program was associated with lower surgical mortality, but we cannot say with confidence that it was due to the program.

continued

TABLE A-2 Continued

Study	Score	Outcome Measures	Measurement Tool	Type of Study	Sample Size
Patterson et al., 2013	IIB	Observed teamwork and communication in both simulated and clinical setting—five observers watched videotapes to assess changes in teamwork behaviors; number of safety events	Clinical database; modified Behavioral Markers for Neonatal Resuscitation Scale	BA	289 in initial training, 151 reevaluated at 10 months; MDs, RNs, RTs, emergency medical technicians (EMTs), patient care assistants (PCAs)
Phipps et al., 2012	IIB	Adverse Outcomes Index—number of deliveries with adverse events; frequency of event reporting; surveys on safety culture	Clinical database, Hospital Survey on Patient Safety Culture (HSPSC)	BA	186 providers at outset = MDs, midwives, RNs, CRNAs, secretaries; number of patients unclear

Setting	Intervention (description)	Findings	Comments (EKP, JKM, VLB)
Academic emergency department	Adapted CRM— initially 12 hours, then reduced to 4 hours.	Significant improvements in teamwork during observed resuscitations—but mostly during simulations. Reduction in safety events.	Actual performance during ED resuscitations assessed; however, only 12 resuscitations observed because of technical limitations of the video recordings. "Individuals participating were frequently acquainted with one another, but intact teams from a particular shift were not trained as a group," yet teamwork and outcomes improved. This is a hopeful finding since teams in practice are often fluid. Total postintervention scores based more on the simulation than on the ED. Only about half of the participants attended the reevaluation at 10 months postintervention. Improvement sustainment is likely biased by the self-selection of participants who completed the reevaluation.
Academic labor and delivery	CRM combined with simulation training.	Improvements in several components of HSPSC. Adverse Outcomes Index declined significantly.	Strong participation with 72 percent of all staff participating (186). But only 120 completed postintervention surveys. Patient data collected at discreet points over time, but only aggregated means used for data analysis.

continued

TABLE A-2 Continued

Study	Score	Outcome Measures	Measurement Tool	Type of Study	Sample Size
Pingleton et al., 2013	IIC	VTE incidence, insertion of peripheral central catheters	Clinical database (chart review)	BA	24 clinicians = MDs, RNs, PharmDs; 261 patients

Setting	Intervention (description)	Findings	Comments (EKP, JKM, VLB)
Academic general acute	An interprofessional, case-based patient safety conference with continuing education (CE) credit was given for physicians, nurses, and pharmacists. Team developed an education plan; a podcast was placed on hospital intranet describing VTE risks; and a patient safety conference was offered for MDs, RNs, and PharmDs. Reference guides were developed and distributed; department data were presented to chairs monthly. A new approach to VTE prophylaxis was approved, and surveillance was enacted. Specific responsibilities for each professional group were developed.	Interdisciplinary team worked together to develop strategic, educational, and system-based plans to decrease incident of VTE. VTE incidence decreased 51 percent. Insertion of peripheral central catheters dropped from almost 360 insertions to fewer than 200 insertions/ month.	The authors selected the highest point over a 4-year period, and compared it with a lower rate toward the end of the study. In fact, the rate at the beginning of the 4-year period was close to the rate at the end. Unclear if the training had any independent impact on outcomes, or it was the simultaneous process changes. This kind of IPE outcome is positive, but interpretation of patient outcomes difficult—i.e., if practice changes were implemented without teamwork in developing them, would the results be the same?

continued

TABLE A-2 Continued

Study	Score	Outcome Measures	Measurement Tool	Type of Study	Sample Size
Sax et al., 2009	IIB	Preoperative checklist use; error self-reporting	Clinical database; OR reports' Web-based error reporting system	BA	857 clinicians trained; MDs, RNs, "ancillary personnel"
Shaw et al., 2014	IIB	Family Satisfaction metrics	Family Satisfaction in the ICU 24 tool (validated)	BA	98 clinicians = MDs, RNs, SWs, chaplains, case managers, PharmDs, RTs; 3 ICUs (36 beds)

Setting	Intervention (description)	Findings	Comments (EKP, JKM, VLB)
Academic and community operating rooms	CRM implemented by outside consulting firm. CME provided to physicians.	Use of a preoperative checklist (developed by a nurse) and incident reporting system improved.	Not clear if CRM training was done with interactive groups and which professions were present in what numbers at each training session. Difficult to say that training had impact on checklist use when "scrub nurse was instructed not to hand up the knife until the checklist was completed," and "any physician who was unwilling to participate was counseled." If the training was simply to empower the nurses to insist on physician compliance, then it was successful, but is this teamwork? Improvements in self-reporting of errors more encouraging.
Community intensive care unit	Self-developed team training program including articles, didactic, simulation, and debriefing.	Multiple measures of family satisfaction with communication improved.	Uncontrolled but interesting study on the effect of training on communication with families.

continued

TABLE A-2 Continued

Study	Score	Outcome Measures	Measurement Tool	Type of Study	Sample Size
Steinemann et al., 2011	IIB	Observed improvements in teamwork during trauma resuscitations; speed and completion of resuscitation; key elements of primary survey and associated labs, time of entry and exit from ED, number and type of procedures, units of blood transfused, avoidable delays to patient transfer	Modified nontechnical skills scale for trauma (T-NOTECHS) (5 teamwork domains, 47 behavioral exemplars done by trained observers during actual resuscitations)	BA	137 team members in 244 blunt trauma resuscitations (141 pre-intervention, 103 post-intervention); MDs, RNs, RTs, ED technicians
Tapson et al., 2011	IIB	Practice: Appropriate administration of VTE prophylaxis to at-risk patients, timing of treatment, duration of treatment inpatient, duration of prophylaxis beyond discharge; Patient: incidence of VTE, readmission rates because of VTE, bleeding events	Review of a random sample of 100 surgical patient charts for listed performance measures both pre- and postintervention	BA	128 providers; 100 patient charts both pre- and post-intervention; MDs, RNs, PharmDs, technicians

Setting	Intervention (description)	Findings	Comments (EKP, JKM, VLB)
Academic emergency department	Human Patient Simulator–based team training (DeVita et al., 2005).	Improvement in mean total T-NOTECHS score, number of teams that completed ≥7 key tasks (out of 8); increased speed and completeness of resuscitation.	Improved scores in simulation and observed actual patient care; measurement of patient outcomes after improvement in team behaviors was documented would have greatly increased the impact of this study.
Community general acute	CRM.	Significant improvement in three performance measures (timing, inpatient duration, and outpatient duration); no difference in patient metrics.	Multiple measures implemented simultaneously. Only 20 percent of those who participated in the preintervention and postintervention confidence surveys continued on and completed the 30-day follow-up. Performance measures were not reported beyond the immediate postintervention period.

continued

TABLE A-2 Continued

Study	Score	Outcome Measures	Measurement Tool	Type of Study	Sample Size
Theilen et al., 2013	IIB	Practice outcomes: time from patient deterioration to clinician response and then to pediatric ICU (PICU) admission; increased frequency of nursing observations, seniority of medical review, patient transfer to high-dependency care prior to PICU admission; Patient outcomes: sickness on admission (PIM2 score), LOS, mortality	Clinical database	BA	Clinicians (not given) = MDs, RNs; patients: 56 preintervention and 54 postintervention
Wolf et al., 2010	IIB	Case delays, case scores: handoff issues, equipment issues/delays, adherence to guidelines for antibiotic administration	Clinical database; definition of "case score" not clear	BA	4,836 surgeries; number of clinicians trained not given; MDs, CRNAs, RNs, technicians

Setting	Intervention (description)	Findings	Comments (EKP, JKM, VLB)
Britain academic intensive care unit	Weekly IPE training (4-10 sessions per year) introduced simultaneously with creation of new pediatric medical emergency team (PMET).	Improvements in time to response, frequency of nursing observations, consultant review, transfer to high-dependency unit, time from first response to PICU admission.	Implemented new PMET structure simultaneously with team training, so impact of training is not clear. Data reported at multiple points pre- and postintervention, but averages used for data analysis. Interestingly, authors include a graphic that shows significant decline in total hospital deaths after introduction of PMETs and training, but documents no significant decline in PICU mortality.
Academic operating room	One-day IPE MTT activity followed by briefing/debriefing protocol for each surgical procedure. Some elements of CRM, some QI training. All elective operations canceled for that day so all could attend.	Significant improvement in delays and case scores and case issues maintained at 2 years.	Large study and results at 1 and 2 years. Represents another study in which team training included planning and implementation of other interventions ("MTT processes" such as debriefings) that then confound analysis of whether the training itself was responsible for outcomes.

continued

TABLE A-2 Continued

Study	Score	Outcome Measures	Measurement Tool	Type of Study	Sample Size
Young-Xu et al., 2011	IIB	Veterans Affairs (VA) Surgical Quality Improvement Program (VASQIP) annual morbidity rates (number of morbidities/ number of procedures); Specifically listed morbidities include DVT, PE, superficial and deep surgical infections; all infections	VASQIP clinical database	BA	74 facilities; 119,383 surgical procedures; "OR teams" (not described)

Setting	Intervention (description)	Findings	Comments (EKP, JKM, VLB)
VHA	VA MTT (communication in the OR and teamwork; checklists, pre- and postoperative briefings) (based on CRM)—high-quality robust training.	Significant decrease in morbidity rate in trained facilities as compared with contemporaneous control group.	Large retrospective cohort study with contemporaneous control group. Self-selection for intervention groups introduces significant bias; used propensity score to minimize this effect. Contemporaneous study group reduces impact of other potential factors, but differences still likely among facilities. Robust training.

Appendix B

Synthesis of Interprofessional Education (IPE) Reviews

Scott Reeves, Ph.D.; Janice Palaganas, Ph.D., R.N., N.P.;
Brenda Zierler, Ph.D., R.N.

INTRODUCTION

In 2010, a review of reviews was published that examined the "meta-evidence" for the effects of interprofessional education (IPE), including changes to collaborative practice and patient care (Reeves et al., 2010). The authors identified 6 IPE reviews published from 2000 to 2008, containing 174 studies. The results indicated that IPE varied in terms of content, duration, and professional participation. It was also found that studies evaluating this form of education were of variable quality and captured a range of different outcomes—from reports of learner satisfaction to changes in the delivery of care. While a number of methodological problems were identified, in general IPE was well-received by learners and enabled the acquisition of knowledge and skills necessary for collaborative work. There was also some evidence suggesting that IPE can improve collaborative practice and the delivery of patient care. To generate an understanding of the latest evidence of the impact of IPE on collaborative practice and patient care, we updated this review of reviews. This latest effort identified eight IPE reviews published from 2010 to 2014, containing 407 studies.[1] The findings from this review of reviews are summarized below in three main sections: methods overview, summary of results, and concluding comments.

---

[1] Although 407 is the total count of included studies from these 8 review papers, it is highly likely that there is multiple reporting of studies in this work due to their overlapping focus. However, it was not possible to identify this overlap because of the limited information contained in the review papers with respect to details of the included studies.

OVERVIEW OF METHODS

To update the 2010 review, we initially searched PubMed for any reviews of IPE published from 2009 to 2014. This search produced 16 published reviews. Each review was assessed independently by the team to determine whether it focused on reporting IPE study outcomes related to collaborative practice and patient care. After this assessment, eight reviews remained.

To help understand the differences among these eight reviews, they were categorized into (1) *systematic reviews* that report directly on included studies, provide detailed information on interprofessional collaboration (IPC)/patient care outcomes, *and* provide methodological quality ratings; and (2) *narrative/scoping reviews*, which provide a more indicative overview of studies, with no formal assessment of the quality of included studies. Based on this categorization, the included reviews were divided into the following groups: *systematic reviews* included Pauze and Reeves (2010) and Reeves et al. (2013); and *scoping/narrative reviews* included Abu-Rish et al. (2012), Brandt et al. (2014), Brody and Galvin (2013), Broyles et al. (2013), Reeves et al. (2011), and Sockalingam et al. (2014).

Steps were then undertaken to analyze and synthesize the evidence contained in the included IPE reviews: (1) familiarization, which entailed a close reading and rereading of reviews to provide an in-depth understanding of the review contents; (2) initial synthesis, which involved a grouping of review data (e.g., search processes, quality assessment techniques, reported outcomes); (3) secondary synthesis, which involved a comparison of research designs and study methodologies used in the reviews to enable an appraisal in these areas; and (4) final synthesis, in which the findings from the previous two steps were combined. This process enabled a critical appraisal and the generation of key synthesized themes.

SUMMARY OF RESULTS

Key results from the synthesis of the included reviews are presented below in two main sections. The first presents general information from the studies included in the systematic and scoping/narrative reviews. The second section presents the key results and describes issues related to the quality of the IPE evidence presented in the reviews.

General Review Information

As noted above and outlined in Table B-1, of the eight included reviews, two were systematic (containing a formal assessment of the quality of included studies), and six were scoping/narrative (providing more descriptive insight into the nature of the included studies).

TABLE B-1 General Review Information

Systematic Reviews			
Review	Details	Methods	Inclusion Criteria
Pauze and Reeves, 2010	Update of 2001 systematic review of the effects of IPE on mental health professionals 16 studies included	Searches: 1999-2007 Medline, CINAHL, PsycInfo Quality: studies scored (1-4) based on assessment of methods, outcomes, and overall clarity of information	Mental health staff involved in delivery of care to adults with mental health issues All research designs included Use of Kirkpatrick outcome typology
Reeves et al., 2013	Update of 2008 systematic review that assessed effectiveness of IPE interventions 9 new studies included (added to 6 studies from 2008 review for a total of 15 studies)	Searches: 2006-2011 Medline, CINAHL, EPOC; reference lists of included papers; manual searches of journals; searches of conference websites Quality: used standard Cochrane criteria to assess quality of included studies	Any IPE intervention Experimental research designs: randomized controlled trial (RCT), controlled before-and-after (CBA) study, and interrupted time series (ITS) study Outcomes: professional practice, patient care, health outcomes, or patient satisfaction
Narrative/Scoping Reviews			
Review	Details	Methods	Inclusion Criteria
Abu-Rish et al., 2012	A narrative review exploring IPE models to identify emerging trends in strategies reported in published studies 83 studies included	Searches: 2005-2010 Pubmed, ISI Web of Knowledge, EMBASE, CINAHL, ERIC, Campbell Collaboration Quality: No assessment of studies undertaken	Qualitative, quantitative, and mixed-methods IPE studies published in peer-reviewed journals All reported IPE outcomes

continued

TABLE B-1 Continued

Review	Details	Methods	Inclusion Criteria
Brandt et al., 2014	A scoping review to determine the success of the IPE/ interprofessional collaboration (IPC) studies in achieving the Triple Aim outcomes 496 papers included. (sub-analysis of 133 research papers)	Searches: 2008-2013 Ovid Medline Quality: No assessment undertaken	Qualitative, quantitative, and mixed-methods studies reporting an IPE/ IPC evaluation Outcomes: studies that reported Triple Aim outcomes
Brody and Galvin, 2013	Systematic review to examine IPE studies reporting patient and provider outcomes related to dementia care 18 articles included (reporting 16 studies)	Searches: 1990-2012 Medline, CINAHL, PsycInfo, and EMBASE Quality: No assessment of studies undertaken	Qualitative, quantitative, and mixed-methods IPE studies reporting dementia intervention Outcomes: health professional knowledge, behavioral changes, or patient outcomes
Broyles et al., 2013	A scoping review to provide an overview of the state of collaboration in addiction education 30 studies included	Searches: 1990-2012 PubMed, Medline, CINAHL, PsychInfo, Google Scholar Quality: No assessment of studies undertaken	Qualitative, quantitative, and mixed-methods IPE studies in the field of addiction education Outcomes related to addiction education
Reeves et al., 2011	Scoping review to help understand clarity of different interprofessional (IP) interventions 104 studies included	Searches: database of IPE studies, Medline, reference lists from IP reviews, manual journal searches Quality: No assessment of studies undertaken	Qualitative, quantitative, and mixed-methods IPE studies published in peer-reviewed journals All reported IPE outcomes

TABLE B-1 Continued

Review	Details	Methods	Inclusion Criteria
Sockalingam et al., 2014	A review aimed at identifying evidence for the value of IPE in delirium programs	Searches: 1965-2013 Medlne, PsychINFO, EMBASE, Web of Science, ERIC, MedEdPortal, BEME	Qualitative, quantitative, and mixed-methods IPE studies involving delirium care
	10 studies located	No quality assessment undertaken	Outcomes: Barr et al. expanded Kirkpatrick typology

NOTE: BEME = Best Evidence Medical Evaluation; CINAHL = Cumulative Index to Nursing and Allied Health Literature; EMBASE = Excerpta Medical Database; EPOC = Effective Practice and Organization of Care; ERIC = Education Resources Information Center; IPE = interprofessional education.

Most of the included reviews shared similar inclusion criteria, which resulted in the inclusion of qualitative, quantitative, and mixed-methods studies. In addition, most employed an expanded Kirkpatrick outcomes typology (Barr et al., 2005), consisting of six different types of outcome (reaction, modification of attitudes/perceptions, acquisition of knowledge/ skills, behavioral change, change in organizational practice, and benefits to patients/clients). Only one of the included reviews was more restrictive, limiting included studies to quantitative designs—randomized controlled trials (RCTs), controlled before-and-after (CBA) studies, and interrupted time series (ITS) studies—and reporting only validated professional practice and health care outcomes.

The range of IPE activities reported in these reviews includes different combinations of professional groups involving different activities and time periods, and delivered in different education and clinical practice settings.

Key Findings and Quality of Evidence

Table B-2 provides an overview of the key results and quality of evidence in the IPE reviews. As indicated in the table, the majority of reviews contain IPE studies that found positive learner-focused outcomes, usually linked to reactions, changes of perception/attitudes, and/or changes in knowledge/skills. Fewer studies found outcomes related to individual behavior. A small proportion of studies in the reviews found positive changes in organizational practice resulting from the delivery of IPE. A smaller number of studies contained in the reviews found changes in the delivery of care to patients/clients, typically in terms of changes in clinical outcomes.

TABLE B-2 Key Review Findings and Quality of Evidence

Systematic Reviews		
Review	Key Findings	Quality of Evidence
Pauze and Reeves, 2010	All studies postlicensure IPE. Range of programs (most centered on small-group activities); outcomes focused on improving team functioning, collaboration, empowering consumers, enhancing integration of services. All but one study report positive outcomes; nine studies report outcomes at level 3, six studies at level 4b, and four studies at level 4a.	Overall improvement in methodological rigor of research designs from the previous 2001 review, with use of more mixed-methods approaches and more complex levels of education outcomes; however, quality of studies still uneven for identifying the effects of IPE for mental health providers. Five studies assessed as "good quality," five studies as "acceptable quality," four studies as "poor quality," and two studies as "unacceptable quality."
Reeves et al., 2013	All studies postlicensure IPE. Seven studies report positive outcomes: diabetes care, emergency department culture and patient satisfaction, collaborative team behaviour and reduction of clinical error rates for emergency department teams, collaborative team behavior in operating rooms, management of care delivered in cases of domestic violence, mental health practitioner competencies for the delivery of patient care. Four studies had mixed (positive and neutral) outcomes; Four studies found IPE had no impact on either professional practice or patient care.	General limitations: small number of studies; heterogeneous IPE interventions, research designs, and outcome measures. The quality of evidence was "low" in the following areas: patient outcomes (six studies), adherence rates to clinical guidelines/standards (three studies), patient satisfaction (two studies), clinical process outcomes (one study). The quality of evidence was "very low" for collaborative behavior (three studies), error rates (one study), practitioner competencies (one study).

TABLE B-2 Continued

Narrative/Scoping Reviews		
Review	Key Findings	Quality of Evidence
Abu-Rish et al., 2012	All studies include IPE outcomes. Sixty-seven studies report more than one outcome. Following outcomes included students' attitudes toward IPE (n = 64), knowledge of collaboration or clinical systems (n = 33), student satisfaction with IPE (n = 30), team skills (n = 25). Patient/clinical outcomes reported in 6 studies, "other" (not specified) outcomes in 30 studies.	No formal assessment of quality undertaken. Authors note a rare use of longitudinal designs and use of surveys (63 studies) and/or interviews/focus groups (37 studies) in most of the included studies.
Brandt et al., 2014	Of 133 research papers included 71 studies based in practice, 42 studies in education, and 14 in mixed setting. Level of analysis for study results: 79 studies report practice-based focus; 28 studies report individual-level knowledge, skills, attitudes focus; 22 studies report organizational-level change. Papers scored for attention to Triple Aim (0 = no Triple Aim outcome; 1 = one outcome; 2 = two outcomes; 3 = all outcomes). 81.2 percent of studies scored 0; 16.5 percent scored 1; 2.3 percent scored 2; none scored 3.	No formal assessment of quality undertaken. Authors note that 67 studies used qualitative methods, 41 quantitative methods, and 24 mixed methods. Approximately 62 percent of the studies report sample sizes of less than 50, and 17 percent report sample sizes of more than 300.

continued

TABLE B-2 Continued

Review	Key Findings	Quality of Evidence
Brody and Galvin, 2013	Based on 16 included studies, authors note that IPE in dementia has potential to provide improved knowledge and attitudes for staff; IPE and structural reform have the potential to improve patient outcomes; IPE interventions that include structural reforms within institutions have the potential to sustain long-term change in practice. Most of the studies were multidisciplinary, not interprofessional in nature.	No formal assessment of quality undertaken. Authors note methodological limitations (i.e., underpowered studies) related to outcome measures in four studies. It is also noted that four studies were sufficiently powered, and that varying methodologies and foci of IPE interventions did not allow for meta-analyses or direct comparison.
Broyles et al., 2013	Based on analysis of 30 studies, reported outcomes are limited to participants' general satisfaction with IPE and/or self-reported confidence/self-efficacy in applying new knowledge and skills. A few studies (numbers not given) report changes in health professionals' and health professional students' substance abuse knowledge. It is noted that only three studies report practice changes.	No formal assessment of quality undertaken. Authors note a lack of conceptual and terminological clarity; wide range of different IPE programs and activities used.

TABLE B-2 Continued

Review	Key Findings	Quality of Evidence
Reeves et al., 2011	One hundred four studies met the criteria and were included for analysis. Studies were examined for their approach to conceptualization, implementation, and assessment of their interprofessional (IP) interventions. Half of the studies were used for IP framework development and half for framework testing and refinement. All studies report some form of "intermediate" outcome (related to the expanded Kirkpatrick typology); 17 studies report changes in patient care; 4 studies report changes in system outcomes (economics).	No formal assessment of quality undertaken. Authors note studies were used to map the literature to identify key concepts, theories, and sources of evidence in order to develop a theoretically based and empirically tested understanding of IPE/ interprofessional collaboration (IPC). Authors note limited use of theory in the studies, so theoretical aspects were not incorporated into the framework. A range of research designs were used, including pre/post (n = 51), poststudy (n = 18), randomized controlled trials (RCTs) (n = 10), and qualitative methods (n = 8). Some mixed methods were used and some longitudinal designs.
Sockalingam et al., 2014	Combined IPE and interprofessional practice (IPP) approach to delirium education can result in higher-order education outcomes (e.g., changes in team behaviors in clinical settings and improved patient outcomes). IPP interventions with higher-level education outcomes are most likely to be associated with interventions that integrate interactive instructional methods and practice-based interventions that are consistent with enabling and reinforcing strategies.	No formal assessment of quality undertaken. Authors note a lack of RCTs and qualitative studies on IP in delirium education resulted in less conclusive recommendations. Expanded Kirkpatrick levels of studies: 1 = two studies; 2a = no studies; 2b = three studies; 3 = six studies; 4a = two studies; 4b = five studies. At the behavior level, two studies self-report an increase in team competence and performance.

Many of the IPE studies in the included reviews contain methodological weaknesses. For example, a number of studies offer only limited or partial descriptions of their IPE programs. Many studies provide little discussion of the methodological limitations of their research. Identification of changes in individual collaborative behavior is particularly poor, often relying on self-reported accounts of this form of change. Most change recorded in the studies was self-reported by learners themselves.

Across the studies, most report the short-term impacts associated with their varying IPE interventions in relation to changes in learner attitudes and knowledge. As a result, understanding of the longer-term impact of IPE on collaborative practice and patient care continues to be limited. Most of the IPE studies contained in the reviews were undertaken at a single site, in isolation from other studies, limiting the generalizability of the research.

Despite a number of weaknesses in the quality of evidence offered by the IPE reviews, there are some encouraging findings in terms of quality. Most notably, there was a fairly common use of quasi-experimental research designs, which can provide some indication of change associated with the delivery of IPE. In addition, most studies included two or more forms of data, and there was continuing use of longitudinal studies to begin to establish the longer-term impact of IPE on organizations and patient care.

CONCLUDING COMMENTS

This work updated a previous synthesis of reviews (Reeves et al., 2010). As indicated above, the evidence for the effects of IPE continues to rest on a variety of different IPE programs (e.g., in terms of learning activities, duration, and professional mix) and evaluation/research methods (experimental studies, mixed methods, qualitative studies) of variable quality. Nevertheless, this updated review of reviews revealed that IPE can nurture collaborative knowledge, skills, and attitudes. It also found more limited, but growing, evidence that IPE can help enhance collaborative practice and improve patient care.

REFERENCES

Abu-Rish, E., S. Kim, L. Choe, L. Varpio, E. Malik, A. A. White, K. Craddick, K. Blondon, L. Robins, P. Nagasawa, A. Thigpen, L. L. Chen, J. Rich, and B. Zierler. 2012. Current trends in interprofessional education of health sciences students: A literature review. *Journal of Interprofessional Care* 26(6):444-451.

Barr, H., I. Koppel, S. Reeves, M. Hammick, and D. Freeth. 2005. *Effective interprofessional education: Argument, assumption, and evidence.* Oxford and Malden, MA: Blackwell Publishing.

Brandt, B., M. N. Lutfiyya, J. A. King, and C. Chioreso. 2014. A scoping review of interprofessional collaborative practice and education using the lens of the triple aim. *Journal of Interprofessional Care* 28(5):393-399.

Brody, A. A., and J. E. Galvin. 2013. A review of interprofessional dissemination and education interventions for recognizing and managing dementia. *Gerontology & Geriatrics Education* 34(3):225-256.

Broyles, L. M., J. W. Conley, J. D. Harding, Jr., and A. J. Gordon. 2013. A scoping review of interdisciplinary collaboration in addictions education and training. *Journal of Addictions Nursing* 24(1):29-36; quiz 37-38.

Pauze, E., and S. Reeves. 2010. Examining the effects of interprofessional education on mental health providers: Findings from an updated systematic review. *Journal of Mental Health (Abingdon, England)* 19(3):258-271.

Reeves, S., J. Goldman, A. Burton, and B. Sawatzky-Girling. 2010. Synthesis of systematic review evidence of interprofessional education. *Journal of Allied Health* 39(Suppl. 1):198-203.

Reeves, S., J. Goldman, J. Gilbert, J. Tepper, I. Silver, E. Suter, and M. Zwarenstein. 2011. A scoping review to improve conceptual clarity of interprofessional interventions. *Journal of Interprofessional Care* 25(3):167-174.

Reeves, S., L. Perrier, J. Goldman, D. Freeth, and M. Zwarenstein. 2013. Interprofessional education: Effects on professional practice and healthcare outcomes (update). *Cochrane Database of Systematic Reviews* 3.

Sockalingam, S., A. Tan, R. Hawa, H. Pollex, S. Abbey, and B. D. Hodges. 2014. Interprofessional education for delirium care: A systematic review. *Journal of Interprofessional Care* 28(4):345-351.

Appendix C

Open Session Agenda

Measuring the Impact of Interprofessional Education (IPE) on
Collaborative Practice and Patient Outcomes: A Consensus Study

October 7, 2014

Keck Center of the National Academies
500 Fifth Street, NW
Washington, DC 20001

STATEMENT OF TASK

An ad hoc committee under the auspices of the Institute of Medicine
(IOM) will examine the methods needed to measure the impact of interprofessional education (IPE) on collaborative practice, patient outcomes,
or both, as determined by the available evidence. Considerable research
on IPE has focused on assessing student learning, but only recently have
researchers begun looking beyond the classroom for impacts of IPE on such
issues as patient safety, provider and patient satisfaction, quality of care,
community health outcomes, and cost savings.

The committee will analyze the available data and information to
determine the best methods for measuring the impact of IPE on specific
aspects of health care delivery and health care systems functioning, such
as IPE impacts on collaborative practice and patient outcomes (including
safety and quality of care). Following review of the available evidence, the

committee will recommend a range of different approaches based on the best available methodologies that measure the impact of IPE on collaborative practice, patient outcomes, or both. The committee will also identify gaps where further research is needed. These recommendations will be targeted primarily at health professional educational leaders.

OPEN SESSION OF CONSENSUS STUDY COMMITTEE (webcast)

SESSION I: LAYING THE FOUNDATION

9:15 am   **Welcome**
Malcolm Cox, Chair

9:30 am   **Views of the Sponsors**
Moderator: Afaf Meleis, Global Forum on Innovation in Health Professional Education Co-Chair
• Maria Tassone, University of Toronto/Canadian Interprofessional Health Leadership Collaborative (CIHLC)
• Carol Aschenbrener, Association of American Medical Colleges/Interprofessional Education Collaborative (IPEC)
• Deborah Trautman, American Association of Colleges of Nursing
Q&A

10:15 am   **The Different Forms and Foci of Interprofessional Education (IPE)**
• Mattie Schmitt, American Academy of Nursing
Q&A

11:00 am   **A Broad Perspective of IPE and Collaborative Practice**
• Hugh Barr, Centre for the Advancement of Interprofessional Education (CAIPE), United Kingdom (joining by phone)
Q&A

11:30 am   **Background Paper**
• Tina Brashers, Author of Background Paper
• Response to Findings: Jill Thistlethwaite, Fellow at the National Center for Interprofessional Practice and Education
Q&A

12:30 pm   **WORKING LUNCH:** Follow-up Questions and Discussion on Background Paper

SESSION II: IMPACTS OF IPE AND COLLABORATION

1:30 pm   **Teamwork and Patient Outcomes**
- Shirley Sonesh, Postdoctoral Research Scientist Working with Eduardo Salas

Q&A with Eduardo Salas (joining by phone)

2:30 pm   **BREAK**

2:45 pm   **Cost of Care and Population Outcomes**
- Stephan Fihn, Patient-Centered Medical Home Demonstration Lab Coordinating Center, Department of Veterans Affairs (virtual connection)

Q&A

SESSION III: METHODOLOGY FOR MEASURING IPE AND COLLABORATION

3:45 pm   **Methodological Implications for Measuring Outcomes of Complex Interactions Like IPE and Interprofessional Practice (IPP)**
- Esther Suter, Workforce Research & Evaluation, Alberta Health Services, Calgary (virtual connection)

Q&A

4:45 pm   **ADJOURNMENT of Open Session**

Appendix D

Global Forum on Innovation in Health Professional Education Sponsors

Academic Consortium for Complementary and Alternative Health Care
Academy of Nutrition and Dietetics
Accreditation Council for Graduate Medical Education
Aetna Foundation
Alliance for Continuing Education in the Health Professions
American Academy of Family Physicians
American Academy of Nursing
American Association of Colleges of Nursing
American Association of Colleges of Osteopathic Medicine
American Association of Colleges of Pharmacy
American Association of Nurse Anesthetists
American Association of Nurse Practitioners
American Board of Family Medicine
American Board of Internal Medicine
American College of Nurse-Midwives
American Congress of Obstetricians and Gynecologists (ACOG)/
    American Board of Obstetrics and Gynecology (ABOG)
American Council of Academic Physical Therapy
American Dental Education Association
American Medical Association
American Occupational Therapy Association
American Psychological Association
American Society for Nutrition
American Speech–Language–Hearing Association
Association of American Medical Colleges

Association of American Veterinary Medical Colleges
Association of Schools and Colleges of Optometry
Association of Schools and Programs of Public Health
Association of Schools of the Allied Health Professions
Atlantic Philanthropies
China Medical Board
Council of Academic Programs in Communication Sciences and Disorders
Council on Social Work Education
Ghent University
Josiah Macy Jr. Foundation
Kaiser Permanente
National Academies of Practice
National Association of Social Workers
National Board for Certified Counselors, Inc. and Affiliates
National Board of Medical Examiners
National League for Nursing
Office of Academic Affiliations of the Veterans Health Administration
Organization of Associate Degree Nursing
Physician Assistant Education Association
Robert Wood Johnson Foundation
Society for Simulation in Healthcare
Uniformed Services University of the Health Sciences
University of Toronto

Appendix E

Speaker Biographies

Carol A. Aschenbrener, M.D., M.S., joined the Association of American Colleges (AAMC) in April 2004, after nearly 30 years as a medical school faculty member and administrator. After serving for 2 years as vice president of the Division of Medical School Standards and Assessments and Liaison Committee on Medical Education (LCME) secretary, she assumed leadership of the Division of Medical Education. In January 2007, she was appointed to the new role of executive vice president and chief strategy officer, and spent nearly 5 years focusing on the implementation of AAMC's strategic priorities and the development of systems to align people and resources with those priorities. In November 2011, she assumed leadership of the newly defined Medical Education Cluster, with the goal of developing and implementing a strategy to facilitate the transformation of medical education toward a true continuum of formation grounded in the health needs of the public. Dr. Aschenbrener has extensive executive experience, including 9 years in various dean's office positions at the University of Iowa College of Medicine and 4 years as chancellor of the University of Nebraska Medical Center. As chancellor, she was responsible for four health colleges; the School of Allied Health; the Graduate Program, University Hospital; and a cancer institute. Before joining AAMC, she spent 7 years as a consultant to academic health centers, focusing on strategic planning, systems redesign, leadership development, and executive coaching. Dr. Aschenbrener has served on a variety of professional and civic boards and has held leadership positions in organized medicine at the state and national levels, including terms as appointed member of the LCME, the Accreditation Committee for Continuing Medical Education, and the Accreditation Committee for

Graduate Medical Education; as elected member of the Iowa Medical Society board, the American Medical Association's (AMA's) Council on Medical Education, and the Educational Commission on Foreign Medical Graduates; and as elected chair of the National Board of Medical Examiners. Her current professional interests include competency-based learning and assessment, interprofessional education (IPE), organizational culture, leadership development, and management of change. Dr. Aschenbrener holds a bachelor of arts degree in psychology from Clarke College in Dubuque, Iowa (1966), and a master of science degree in neuroanatomy from the University of Iowa (1968). She received her M.D. degree from the University of North Carolina (1971) and completed residency training in anatomic pathology and neuropathology at the University of Iowa Hospitals and Clinics (1974).

Hugh Barr, M.Phil., Ph.D., is an emeritus editor for the *Journal of Interprofessional Care* and holds visiting chairs in IPE at Curtin in Western Australia and Kingston with St. George's University of London, Greenwich and Suffolk in the United Kingdom. He served on the World Health Organization (WHO) study group on IPE and collaborative practice and until recently convened the World Interprofessional Education and Collaborative Practice Coordinating Committee. Dr. Barr was awarded honorary doctorates by East Anglia and Southampton universities for his role in promoting IPE nationally and internationally.

Valentina Brashers, M.D., FACP, FNAP, is the founder and co-director of the University of Virginia Center for Academic Strategic Partnerships for Interprofessional Research and Education (Center for ASPIRE), which provides leadership and oversight to more than 25 IPE experiences for students, clinicians, and faculty at all levels of training. She is known nationally for her service and scholarship in the area of IPE and collaborative care. She served for many years as vice president for interdisciplinary care for the National Academies of Practice, where she received the Nicholas Cummings Award for Contributions to the Interprofessional Healthcare Field. Dr. Brashers currently is a co–principal investigator for numerous intra- and extramural IPE grants and serves as a consultant, editor, expert panel member, presenter, and workshop leader in many educational, clinical, and policy settings.

Stephan D. Fihn, M.D., M.P.H., FACP, is a general internist and serves as director of the Office of Analytics and Business Intelligence (ABI) in the Veterans Health Administration (VHA) and as a staff physician at the U.S. Department of Veterans Affairs (VA) Puget Sound Health Care System (VAPSHCS). ABI is responsible for analytics and reporting of clinical, operational, and financial data for the VA health system, which provides care to more than 6 million veterans. Dr. Fihn received his medical training at St. Louis University and completed an internship, residency, and chief residency in the Department of Medicine at the University of Washington (UW). He was a Robert Wood Johnson Foundation Clinical Scholar and earned a master's degree in public health at UW, where he has been on the faculty since 1979 and presently holds the rank of professor in the departments of Medicine and of Health Services. From 1993 to 2011, Dr. Fihn directed the Northwest VA Health Services Research & Development Center of Excellence at VAPSHCS. His research has addressed a broad range of topics related to strategies for improving the efficiency and quality of primary medical care and understanding the epidemiology of common medical problems. He received the VA Undersecretary's Award for Outstanding Contributions in Health Services Research in 2002. He served as acting chief research and development officer for the VA in 2004-2005. Dr. Fihn has always striven to apply the principles and findings of health services research to health care delivery. He served as chief quality and performance officer for the VHA, 2007-2008. In his current position, he is responsible for supporting high-level analytics and the delivery of clinical and business information throughout the VA health system. He remains an active clinician and was named a "Top Doc" by *Seattle Metropolitan Magazine* in 2011. He co-edited two editions of a textbook titled *Outpatient Medicine*. Dr. Fihn is active in several academic organizations, including the Society of General Internal Medicine (SGIM) (past-president), the American College of Physicians (fellow), the American Heart Association (fellow), and AcademyHealth. In 2012, he received the Robert J. Glaser Award for outstanding contributions to research, education, or both in generalism in medicine from SGIM.

Afaf I. Meleis, Ph.D., Dr.P.S.(hon), FAAN, has demonstrated a profound passion for pushing the boundaries of nursing science, cultivating the next generation of health care leaders, and improving women's health, over the course of more than five decades. During her tenure as the fifth Dean of the University of Pennsylvania School of Nursing (2002-2014), she fostered a community that is voiced, empowered, and dedicated to making an impact on global healthcare; launched multidisciplinary and global partnerships that are advancing nursing science, education, and practice; expanded research in critical areas; cultivated a culture of innovation where new programs and technologies are being developed to address emerging healthcare challenges; and strengthened its commitment to serving and supporting the local community. Prior to coming to Penn, she was a professor on the faculty of nursing at the University of California, Los Angeles, and the University of California, San Francisco, for 34 years.

Eduardo Salas, Ph.D., is trustee chair and Pegasus professor of psychology at the University of Central Florida (UCF). He also holds an appointment as program director for the Human Systems Integration Research Department at UCF's Institute for Simulation & Training. Previously, he was a senior research psychologist and head of the Training Technology Development Branch of the Naval Air Warfare Center-Orlando for 15 years. During this period, he served as a principal investigator for numerous R&D programs focusing on teamwork, team training, simulation-based training, decision making under stress, learning methodologies, and performance assessment. Dr. Salas has co-authored more than 489 journal articles and book chapters and has co-edited more than 25 books. He is on/has been on the editorial boards of numerous journals. He is past editor of *Human Factors* journal and current associate editor for the *Journal of Applied Psychology* and *Military Psychology*. Dr. Salas has held numerous positions in the Human Factors and Ergonomics Society (HFES) during the past 15 years. He is also very active with the Society for Industrial and Organizational Psychology (SIOP)—Division 14 of the American Psychological Association (APA). He is past president of SIOP and past series editor of the Organizational Frontier and the Professional Practice Book Series. Dr. Salas is a fellow of the APA, the HFES, and the Association for Psychological Science. He received the 2012 Joseph E. McGrath Lifetime Achievement Award for the study of teams and groups from INGroup, the SIOP's 2012 Distinguished Professional Contributions Award, and the 2012 Michael R. Losey Award from the Society for Human Resources Management for his applied contributions to understanding teams and groups as well as training effectiveness. He received his Ph.D. degree (1984) in industrial and organizational psychology from Old Dominion University.

Madeline Schmitt, Ph.D., R.N., FAAN, FNAP, professor emerita, is a nurse-sociologist who, until retirement, was professor and independence foundation chair in nursing and interprofessional education at the University of Rochester (New York) School of Nursing. She remains active in research and publication, as well as limited teaching on interprofessional collaboration. She consults and presents nationally and internationally on the topic. Since the 1970s, she has focused her career on interprofessional collaborative practice models and IPE. Her work with collaborative practice came first, and involved training and teaching about interprofessional clinical teams, as well as research. She was co-investigator on a recently completed National Institutes of Health–funded 4-year ethnography study focused on the incorporation of a palliative care team into the hospital environment. In the IPE arena, Dr. Schmitt was part of a multisite national project co-sponsored by the Institute for Healthcare Improvement and Health Resources and Services Administration (HRSA): Community-based Quality

Improvement Education for the Health Professions. She was the local co–principal investigator for testing the RWJF-funded *Achieving Competency Today* interprofessional quality improvement curriculum. She was one of two U.S. members of the WHO Task Force that produced the report *Framework for Action in Interprofessional Education and Collaborative Practice*. In 2010-2011, Dr. Schmitt chaired an expert panel commissioned by the Interprofessional Education Collaborative (IPEC) to develop U.S. core competencies for interprofessional collaborative practice. The *Core Competencies for Interprofessional Collaborative Practice* report and that of a meeting held to develop action plans for implementation of the core competencies were both released in Washington, DC, at the National Press Club. Dr. Schmitt is an editor emerita of the *Journal of Interprofessional Care* and a founding board member of the American Interprofessional Health Collaborative. She is sole or co-author of more than 100 professional publications, many focused on interprofessional collaboration topics. Her multiple honors include induction as a fellow of the American Academy of Nursing in 1977 and the National Academies of Practice in 2000, which honored her with its Award for Interdisciplinary Creativity.

Shirley Sonesh, Ph.D., is a research scientist at the Institute of Simulation and Training (IST) at UCF. She obtained her doctorate in organizational behavior at A.B. Freeman School of Business at Tulane University. At UCF, Dr. Sonesh leads a team of researchers investigating the effects of medical team training, the effects of telemedicine on teamwork in emergency management situations, simulation-based team training, and the role of IPE in patient outcomes, among many other health care–related initiatives. Dr. Sonesh also consults with organizations on how to improve teamwork in interprofessional medical teams to enhance patient safety. She is a member of the advisory board of Meditel360, a telemedicine firm specializing in home-based care. She has co-authored a number of published articles in the fields of medical team training, training evaluation, translational medical teams, and simulation in health care. Dr. Sonesh has been invited to a number of international and national conferences to present research related to these fields. She is a member of SIOP, Academy of Management (AOM), Society for Simulation in Healthcare (SSH), and American Telehealth Association (ATA).

Esther Suter, Ph.D., M.S.W., is the director of workforce research and evaluation at Alberta Health Services. She holds a Ph.D. in natural sciences (1990) from the Swiss Institute of Technology and an M.S.W. (2003) from the University of Calgary. She has been a health researcher for more than 20 years. Being situated in a provincial health authority allows Dr. Suter to conduct in-depth examination of health systems issues and applied "real-life" research. The focus of her research is on interventions to enhance collaborative practice, how to achieve integrated health systems, and innovative care delivery models. Dr. Suter is or has been the principal investigator on numerous research projects. She has more than 70 publications in peer-reviewed journals.

Maria Tassone, M.Sc., is the inaugural director of the Centre for Interprofessional Education, a strategic partnership between the University of Toronto and the University Health Network (UHN). She is also the senior director, health professions and interprofessional care and integration at the UHN in Toronto, a network of four hospitals comprising Toronto General, Toronto Western, Toronto Rehab, and Princess Margaret. Ms. Tassone holds a bachelor of science degree in physical therapy from McGill University and a master of science degree from the University of Western Ontario, and she is an assistant professor in the Department of Physical Therapy, Faculty of Medicine, University of Toronto. She was the UHN project lead for the coaching arm of Catalyzing and Sustaining Communities of Collaboration around Interprofessional Care, which was recently awarded the Ontario Hospital Association's international Ted Freedman Award for Education Innovation. Her graduate work and scholarly interests focus on continuing education, professional development, and knowledge translation in the health professions. She is the former co-chair of the Canadian Interprofessional Health Collaborative Education Committee, and is currently the lead on the Collaborative Change Leadership program. Throughout her career, Ms. Tassone has held a variety of clinical, education, research, and leadership positions, both within physical therapy and across a multitude of professions. She is most passionate about the interface among research, education, and practice and about leading change in complex systems.

Jill Thistlethwaite, M.B.B.S., Ph.D., M.M.Ed., FRCGP, FRACGP, is a health professions education consultant and practicing family physician in Sydney, Australia. She is currently a Fulbright senior scholar at the National Center for Interprofessional Practice and Education. Dr. Thistlethwaite is affiliated with the University of Technology, Sydney (UTS), the University of Queensland, and Auckland University of Technology (New Zealand). Born in the United Kingdom, she received her medical degree from the University of London and was a general practitioner in a semirural practice in the north of England for 12 years. She became an academic medical educator in 1996, and subsequently obtained her master's degree in medical education from the University of Dundee and her Ph.D. in shared decision making and medical education from the University of Maastricht. Dr. Thistlethwaite's major interests are IPE, communication skills, and professionalism. She has written a book on values-based interprofessional collaboration and co-authored four books and co-edited four—the most recent being two volumes on leadership development for IPE and collaborative practice. She has also published more than 90 peer-reviewed papers and book chapters. Dr. Thistlethwaite has been invited to consult and run workshops on IPE and collaborative practice in Finland, Germany, Indonesia, Malaysia, New Zealand, Singapore, and Switzerland. She has been involved with three major grant programs in Australia focusing on these topics. As co-editor of *The Clinical Teacher* and associate editor of the *Journal of Interprofessional Care,* she is heavily involved in editing and mentoring writers from many countries and of many levels of experience.

Deborah E. Trautman, Ph.D., R.N., assumed the role of Chief Executive Officer of the American Association of Colleges of Nursing (AACN) in June 2014. At AACN, she oversees all of the strategic initiatives, signature programming, and advocacy efforts led by the organization known as the national voice for baccalaureate and graduate nursing education. Formerly the executive director of the Center for Health Policy and Healthcare Transformation at Johns Hopkins Hospital, Dr. Trautman has held clinical and administrative leadership positions at the University of Pittsburgh Medical Center and the Johns Hopkins Medical Institutions. She also served as the Vice President of Patient Care Services for Howard County General Hospital, part of the Johns Hopkins Health System; and as director of Nursing for Emergency Medicine at the Johns Hopkins Hospital. She also held a joint appointment at the Johns Hopkins University School of Nursing. Dr. Trautman received a B.S.N. from West Virginia Wesleyan College, an M.S.N. with emphasis on education and administration from the University of Pittsburgh, and a Ph.D. in health policy from the University of Maryland, Baltimore County. She has authored and coauthored publications on health policy, intimate partner violence, pain management, clinical competency, change management, cardiopulmonary bypass, the use of music in the emergency department, and consolidating emergency services. As a member of the senior leadership at the Johns Hopkins Hospital, she represented the hospital on the Baltimore City Domestic Violence Fatality Review Team. Dr. Trautman serves as an advisory board member and chair for Academy Health's Interdisciplinary Research Interest Group on Nursing Issues. She has served as a Magnet Appraiser Fellow for the American Nurses Association Credentialing Center Commission on Accreditation and as an advisory committee member for the navigator and enrollment committee of the Maryland Health Insurance Exchange. Dr. Trautman is a 2007/2008 RWJF Health Policy Fellow who worked for the Honorable Nancy Pelosi, then Speaker of the House, U.S. House of Representatives.

Appendix F

Committee Member Biographies

Malcolm Cox, M.D. (*Chair*), is an adjunct professor at the Perelman School of Medicine, University of Pennsylvania. He most recently served for 8 years as chief academic affiliations officer for the U.S. Department of Veterans Affairs (VA) in Washington, DC, where he oversaw the largest health professions training program in the country and repositioned the VA as a major voice in clinical workforce reform, education innovation, and organizational transformation. Dr. Cox received his undergraduate education at the University of the Witwatersrand and his M.D. from Harvard Medical School. After completing postgraduate training in internal medicine and nephrology at the Hospital of the University of Pennsylvania, he rose through the ranks to become professor of medicine and associate dean for clinical education at the Perelman School of Medicine. He also served as dean for medical education at Harvard Medical School; upon leaving the Dean's Office, he was appointed Carl W. Walter distinguished professor of medicine at Harvard Medical School. Dr. Cox was the first Robert G. Petersdorf scholar in residence at the Association of American Medical Colleges and has also served on the National Leadership Board of the Veterans Health Administration, the VA National Academic Affiliations Council, the National Board of Medical Examiners, the National Advisory Committee of the Robert Wood Johnson Foundation (RWJF) Clinical Scholars Program, the Board of Directors of the Accreditation Council for Graduate Medical Education, and the Global Forum on Innovation in Health Professional Education of the Institute of Medicine (IOM).

Barbara F. Brandt, Ph.D., is renowned for her work in health professional education, and specifically in interprofessional education (IPE) and continuing education. Dr. Brandt serves as associate vice president for education within the University of Minnesota's Academic Health Center, and she is responsible for the university's *1Health* initiative, aimed at building the interprofessional practice skills of students and faculty in a broad range of health professions. She is also director of the National Center for Interprofessional Practice and Education, a public–private partnership and cooperative agreement with the Health Resources and Services Administration, established in 2012. In her leadership roles, Dr. Brandt has served as a consultant, advisor, and speaker for a wide variety of organizations, such as the IOM, the National Quality Forum, the Academy of Healthcare Improvement, the Josiah Macy Jr. Foundation, the Association of Schools of Allied Health Professions, the American Speech–Language–Hearing Association, and the American Medical Association. She holds a bachelor of arts degree in the teaching of history from the University of Illinois at Chicago and master of education and doctor of philosophy degrees in continuing education (specializing in continuing professional education for the health professions) from the University of Illinois at Urbana-Champaign. In 2013 she was recognized as a University of Illinois distinguished alumna. She completed a W.K. Kellogg Foundation–sponsored postdoctoral fellowship for faculty in adult and continuing education at the University of Wisconsin–Madison.

Janice Palaganas, Ph.D., R.N., N.P., is a lecturer at the Harvard Medical School and director for educational innovation and development for the Institute for Medical Simulation in Boston, Massachusetts—the Center for Medical Simulation's international program for IPE simulation educator training. Dr. Palaganas is a recognized leader and expert in the field of IPE simulation through such activities as serving as the implementing director of the Society for Simulation in Healthcare's (SSH's) Simulation Center Accreditation and Educator Certification Programs, editor-in-chief of SSH's first resource textbook, chair of the 2011 Simulation and IPE Symposium, and founding chair of the SSH IPE Affinity Group. As a behavioral scientist, Dr. Palaganas's passion is in using health care simulation as a platform for IPE, with a strong professional commitment to developing IPE simulation educators. At various times in her career, she has taught for schools of medicine, nursing, pharmacy, allied health, business, religion, and emergency residency, and thus is one of the country's most experienced instructors providing simulation-enhanced IPE to multiple levels of pre- and postlicensure learners. Dr. Palaganas has been a featured or keynote speaker at international and national conferences, and is an author for the National League for Nursing (NLN) study on using simulation-based high-stakes assessment for nursing students and evaluating the challenges of assessing teamwork in simulation. She has also served on the Board of Examiners for the Malcolm Baldrige National Quality Award under the National Institute of Standards and Technology. Dr. Palaganas attended the University of Pennsylvania and there received her bachelor of science degree in nursing, as well as two master's degrees in the fields of advanced practice nursing. She earned her Ph.D. in nursing at Loma Linda University. Prior to her academic career, Dr. Palaganas had wide experience clinically in three different hospital systems as a leader and clinician and held multiple roles in emergency departments. Prior to joining the Harvard Medical School faculty and the Center for Medical Simulation, she served as a Medical Simulation Department chief operations officer and director of simulation research at Loma Linda University. Dr. Palaganas has taught for schools of medicine, nursing, pharmacy, allied health, business, religion, and emergency residency.

Scott Reeves, Ph.D., is a social scientist who has been involved in health professions education and health services research for 20 years. He is a professor in interprofessional research at the Faculty of Health, Social Care & Education, Kingston University & St George's, University of London, and editor-in-chief, *Journal of Interprofessional Care*. Most recently, he was founding director, Center for Innovation in Interprofessional Education; professor of social and behavioral sciences; and professor of medicine, University of California, San Francisco. Previously, he was inaugural director of research, Centre for Faculty Development, St Michael's Hospital, Canada. He also held positions as senior scientist, Wilson Centre for Research in Education, and professor of psychiatry, University of Toronto. During this time he was appointed inaugural evaluation director, Canadian Interprofessional Health Collaborative. Dr. Reeves has also held honorary faculty positions in a number of institutions around the world. His main interests are in developing conceptual, empirical, and theoretical knowledge to inform the design and implementation of IPE and practice activities. To date, he has received more than $18 million in grant capture from a range of funding bodies across the world. He has published more than 250 peer-reviewed papers, book chapters, textbooks, editorials, and monographs; many of his publications have been translated from English into other languages. Dr. Reeves has a long history of national and international committee work. Currently, he is an appointed board member for the UK Centre for the Advancement of Interprofessional Education and a member of the Global Forum on Innovation in Health Professional Education of the IOM. He also has worked on committees for a number of organizations in Canada, the United Kingdom, and the United States. He has received a number of awards for his interprofessional teaching and mentorship.

Albert W. Wu, M.D., M.P.H., is professor of health policy and management and medicine, with joint appointments in epidemiology, international health, medicine, and surgery. He received B.A. and M.D. degrees from Cornell University, and completed an internal medicine residency at the Mount Sinai Hospital and the University of California, San Diego. He was an RWJF clinical scholar at the University of California, San Francisco, and received an M.P.H. degree from the University of California, Berkeley. Dr. Wu's research and teaching focus on patient outcomes and quality of care. He was the first to measure the quality-of-life impact of antiretroviral therapy in HIV clinical trials. He developed the Medical Outcomes Study HIV Health Survey (MOS-HIV) and other questionnaires used to measure quality of life, adherence, satisfaction, attitudes, and behaviors for people with chronic disease. Dr. Wu was co-founder and director of the Outcomes Research Committee of the AIDS Clinical Trials Group of the National Institutes of Health and president of the International Society for Quality of Life. He advises many U.S. and international organizations on patient-reported outcomes (PROs) methods. He is director of the Johns Hopkins Center for Health Services and Outcomes Research and director of the Agency for Healthcare Research and Quality–funded DEcIDE center for patient-centered outcomes research. He is a Patient Reported Outcomes Measurement Information System (PROMIS) investigator, and co-developer of PatientViewpoint, a patient portal used to link patient-reported outcomes to electronic health records. Dr. Wu has studied the handling of medical errors since 1988 and has published influential papers, including "Do House Officers Learn from Their Mistakes" in the *Journal of the American Medical Society* in 1991, and "Medical Error: The Second Victim" in the *British Medical Journal*. He was a member of the IOM committee on identifying and preventing medication errors and was senior adviser for patient safety to the World Health Organization in Geneva. He has authored more than 350 peer-reviewed publications and was editor of the Joint Commission book *The Value of Close Calls in Improving Patient Safety*. He leads the Ph.D. program in health services research and the certificate program in quality, patient safety, and outcomes research in the Johns Hopkins Bloomberg School of Public Health. Dr. Wu maintains a clinical practice in general internal medicine.

Brenda Zierler, Ph.D., R.N., F.A.A.N., explores the relationships between the delivery of health care and outcomes at both the patient and system levels. Her primary appointment is in the School of Nursing at the University of Washington (UW), but she holds three adjunct appointments—two in the School of Medicine and one in the School of Public Health. Currently, Dr. Zierler is co–principal investigator on a Josiah Macy Jr. Foundation–funded grant with Dr. Les Hall, focused on developing a national train-the-trainer faculty development program for IPE and collaborative practice. She also leads two Health Resources and Services Administration training grants—one focusing on technology-enhanced IPE for advanced practice students and the second on interprofessional collaborative practice for advanced heart failure patients at UW's Regional Heart Center. Dr. Zierler is the co-director for the UW Center for Health Sciences Interprofessional Education, Practice and Research, as well as director of faculty development for the UW Institute for Simulation and Interprofessional Studies in the School of Medicine. She is a board member and chair of the American Interprofessional Health Collaborative and a member of the IOM Global Forum on Innovation in Health Professional Education.